Companion Animal Economics

The Economic Impact of Companion Animals in the UK

Research Report

Companion Animal Economics

The Economic Impact of Companion Animals in the UK

Research Report

Sophie Hall,[1] Luke Dolling,[2] Katie Bristow,[3] Ted Fuller[2] and Daniel Mills[1]

[1]*School of Life Sciences, University of Lincoln, UK*
[2]*Lincoln Business School, University of Lincoln, UK*
[3]*Dogs for Good, Banbury, UK*

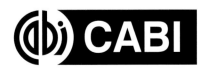

CABI is a trading name of CAB International

CABI
Nosworthy Way
Wallingford
Oxfordshire OX10 8DE
UK

CABI
745 Atlantic Avenue
8th Floor
Boston, MA 02111
USA

Tel: +44 (0)1491 832111
Fax: +44 (0)1491 833508
E-mail: info@cabi.org
Website: www.cabi.org

Tel: +1 (617)682-9015
E-mail: cabi-nao@cabi.org

A catalogue record for this book is available from the British Library, London, UK.

Library of Congress Cataloging-in-Publication Data

Names: Hall, Sophie (Sophie Susannah), author. | Dolling, Luke, author. | Bristow, Katie, author. | Fuller, Ted (Professor of entrepreneurship and strategic foresight), author. | Mills, D. S., author. | C.A.B. International, publisher.
Title: Companion animal economics : the economic impact of companion animals in the UK : research report / Sophie Hall, Luke Dolling, Katie Bristow, Ted Fuller, Daniel Mills.
Description: Wallingford, Oxfordshire ; Boston, MA : CABI, [2017] | Includes bibliographical references and index.
Identifiers: LCCN 2016041649 (print) | LCCN 2016043081 (ebook) | ISBN 9781786391728 (pbk. : alk. paper) | ISBN 9781786391735 (pdf) | ISBN 9781786391742 (ePub)
Subjects: | MESH: Bonding, Human-Pet | Pets--economics | Pets--psychology | Health | Great Britain
Classification: LCC SF411.36.G7 (print) | LCC SF411.36.G7 (ebook) | NLM WM 460.5.B7 | DDC 636.088/70941--dc23
LC record available at https://lccn.loc.gov/2016041649

ISBN-13: 978 1 78639 172 8

Commissioning editor: Caroline Makepeace
Associate editor: Alexandra Lainsbury
Production editor: Tracy Head

Typeset by SPi, Pondicherry, India.
Printed and bound by Gutenberg Press Ltd, Tarxien, Malta.

Contents

This book is enhanced with supplementary resources. To access the Appendix
Tables, please visit: www.cabi.org/openresources/91728.

Foreword

The relationship between people and pets is a unique bond that has endured over many centuries. Almost half of households in the UK share their homes with animals cared for as companions; a relationship we consider to be valuable, enriching, mutually beneficial and fun. Because we share our lives with companion animals in such close proximity, we each impact the other. Increasingly, scientific evidence suggests that companion animals bring social, health and economic benefits to individuals and society.

This report was inspired by the seminal Council for Science and Society report *Companion Animals in Society*, published in 1988, which provided a clear view of the role of companion animals in Britain, including an exploration of the economic impact of pets. The world has changed since the late eighties: we now have an increasingly urban and aged population, with smaller and more fragmented families. Despite this, relatively little information on the economic impact of pets has been published since 1988. This important report provides a modern day update and, without reducing the discussion to a simplistic cost:benefit ratio, it includes new data from the myriad of ways in which companion animals contribute to our society in the UK, as well as some of the costs they bring.

This report aims to raise awareness of the important need for research to evaluate the complex routes by which pets make an economic impact on UK society. It aims to dispel the myth that pets are a luxury and to increase awareness of the social, economic and health value of pets to society so that better informed debate and decisions can be made for the benefit of people and pets.

Dr Sandra McCune
WALTHAM Centre for Pet Nutrition
Leicestershire, UK

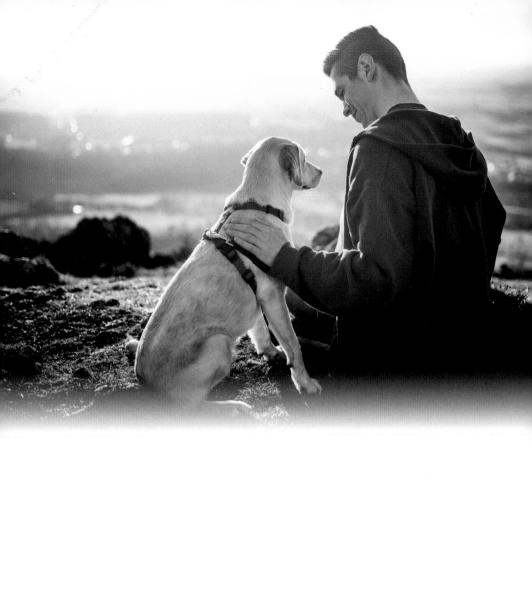

Executive Summary

- The aim of this report is to raise awareness of the importance of research concerning the economic impact of companion animals on society.
- This report was inspired by the seminal Council for Science and Society (CSS) report *Companion Animals in Society* (1988), and updates and extends its evaluation of the value that companion animals bring to society.
- Data available from the UK are used as examples throughout, but many of the points raised relate to industrialized nations globally.
- It highlights potential direct and indirect costs and benefits of companion animals to the economy, and the value of exploring these further.
- There is currently a lack of high quality data for some aspects of this evaluation which needs to be addressed to enable a more confident analysis; however, given the scale of the potential impact (added economic value and savings possible) the matter should not be ignored for this reason.
- When evaluating the contribution of companion animals to the UK economy both positive and negative aspects should be considered.
- Employing a conservative version of methods used in the best study of its kind to date examining healthcare savings through reduced number of doctor visits, we estimate that pet ownership in the UK may reduce use of the National Health Service (NHS) to the value of £2.45 billion/year.
- The cost of NHS treatment for bites and strikes from dogs is estimated as £3 million/year (i.e. approximately 0.1% of the health savings).
- We conclude that research into companion animals that relates to their potential economic impact on society should be supported by government.

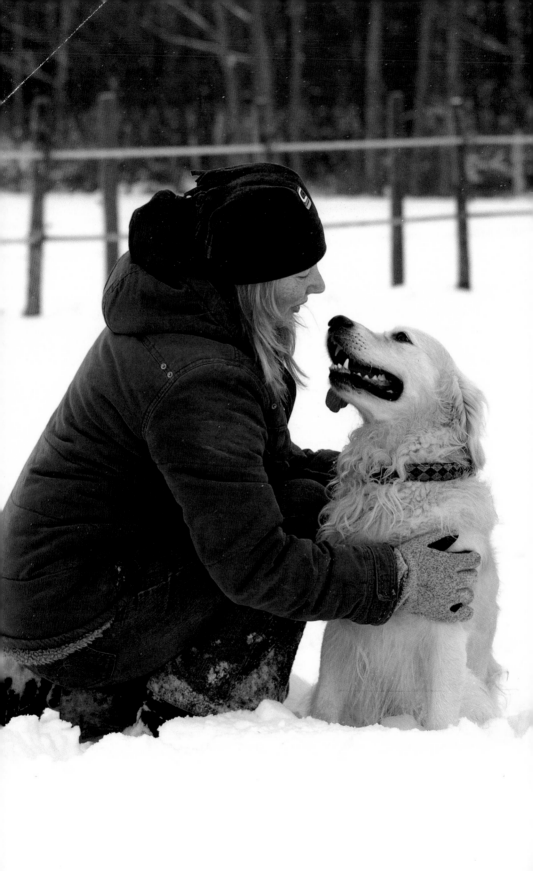

Introduction

The UK is renowned as being a nation of animal lovers, with an estimated 12 million (46%) households incorporating about 65 million companion animals into their families (PFMA, 2015). With close proximity comes an opportunity to impact on each other's health and well-being. More broadly, it reflects a societal impact. The scale of this phenomenon raises the need for insight into the extent to which we share our lives with companion animals, and the nature of the human–animal relationship in these contexts. Indeed, human society is inherently multispecies (Mills & De Keuster, 2009).

In this report we wish to highlight the economic significance especially of the *companionship* of animals and use the term '**companion animal**' to refer to those animals (e.g. dogs and cats) that keep us company in a range of contexts. This recognizes the animal's family member status in Western traditions as well as acknowledging its individuality, and the compatibility of bonds within the relationship. It could be argued that domestic equids fall into this category, but these are beyond the scope of this report. Even within *companion animal* species, the boundaries are indistinct; for example many working dogs (animals employed to work with a handler in a specific type or range of tasks, such as police and security dogs and working gun dogs) are no longer viewed as important for just their instrumental value, but are of increasingly important emotional value to their handlers, who may work in very stressful conditions. This is particularly the case with assistance animals (animals kept to provide help or assistance to those who are not fully able bodied such as guide dogs or assistance dogs). While it is appropriate to acknowledge the additional economic value of these animals in terms of the work they do, quantifying this value is beyond the scope of this report. Nonetheless, we have tried to scope the demographics of these populations in some of the appendices and include the health benefits of assistance animals as a special case for consideration given that their production is based on the charitable rather than governmental or commercial sectors. We tend to avoid the term '**pet**' since this implies a somewhat unidirectional, utilitarian relationship, in which the animal is largely a possession of its keeper, kept for the pleasure that the relationship brings that individual (e.g. pet dog). However, we retain the term 'pet' as an adjective where it is commonly used (e.g. 'pet food' and 'pet shop'). Companion animals are often considered valuable members of the community, for many different reasons, depending on the role they fulfil. Nonetheless, we also recognize that this is not without a potential cost as well. Where possible we have provided figures relating to these in the supplementary tables. However, the primary aim of this report is to recognize the differing roles that companion animals have within our society and to explore the *possible value* that they bring through these roles, in an economic sense, so the narrative predominantly focuses on their contribution to society. Indeed, the economic contribution of companion animals to society is reported to be growing annually, despite the current economic downturn. There is increased availability of ever more products and services for animal companions, but also a greater need for the psychological and physical benefits they can bring during times of hardship.

This report serves as a preliminary examination of the scope and extent of the economic value of companion animals within the UK. It is to be hoped that not only will the report act as a point of reference for contextualizing this important function, but also that it will serve as a basis for further refinement and monitoring in the future. The analysis encompasses numerous strands, some of which are more readily measured than others. The scope includes the contribution of the economic impact of the pet care industry, the reported health and well-being benefits of companion animal ownership and the value of working animals in their various roles in society. It is important to note that the 'role in society' and 'social value' of companion animals are not fixed phenomena but change over time and situation. Indeed, there has seemingly been a shift from objectification to subjectification of companion animals within society in recent years; they are seen less as chattels or possessions and more as individuals in their own right, and as members of the family. This might reflect a shift in our emotional bond with them and our perceptions as a consequence.

The roles that companion animal species are given within our society range from: pets to working animals, leisure performers (e.g. in sport), assistance animals, service animals (e.g. police, military, fire, search and rescue) and laboratory subjects. These categories are neither rigid nor exclusive, but can merge and change over time. For example, while the assistance dog partnered with a person to provide practical support may be perceived by some primarily as a working animal, the owner may well value the dog's companionship in higher regard than the support or assistance he or she was originally sourced for.

Specifically, this report aims to help to dispel the myth that companion animals are a decadent luxury, and to increase awareness of the social, economic and health impact of companion animals on society, so that better informed debate and decisions can be made for the benefit of society.

Methodology

2

This preliminary study was a desk-based research exercise, inspired by the seminal Council for Science and Society (CSS) report *Companion Animals in Society* (1988), which was the starting point for the investigation.

The CSS report (1988) attempted to produce a comprehensive evaluation of the significance of companion animals in the UK, providing a benchmark for discussing their economic impact within our society. At the time, the report was seemingly presented as the only report to attempt such an evaluation, with no updates since 1988.

Content analysis and deconstruction of the CSS report was undertaken to elicit core concepts, repeating themes and underpinning assumptions. Specific attention was placed on economic data and figures relating to companion animals and society. Data and figures presented in the original report were extracted and tabulated, with the original assumption and/or references for such figures also noted. Through collection of such data, an attempt was made to source more recent figures giving a revised overview of the economic impact of companion animals.

The context of companion animals in society and the associated industries has changed in the last 25–30 years, and therefore further economic considerations were also generated that were not included in the CSS report. Such considerations included UK companion animal-related exports and imports, further industry employment information, the impact of companion animals in the workplace, the impact of national trends like an economic downturn on the perceived value of companion animals, pet tourism, expanding veterinary services, new companion animal services and functions, development of animal welfare charities (i.e. number of volunteers and revenue) and companion animal advertising. Where it was easily available, comparable data and analyses from other countries were accessed, to help provide benchmarks and context for the UK data.

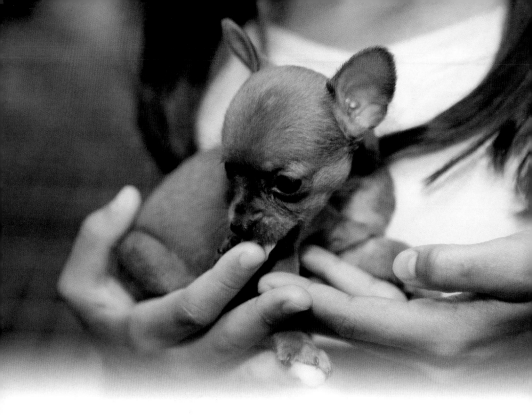

Techniques Revisited and Updated

Within the CSS report it was found that a relatively small number of sources were used for figures provided. Sources given included organizations such as: the British Horse Society, the Kennel Club, the Pet Trade and Industry Association, the Governing Council of the Cat Fancy (GCCF), the National Exhibition of Cage and Aviary Birds, the British Federation of Aquarists, the Union of Communication Workers and the Post Office. Charitable organizations were also identified, including The Guide Dogs for the Blind Association and Pro-dogs. Further sources encompassed the Yellow Pages™, miscellaneous other studies and reports, a small number of academic articles, as well as estimates from a London wholesaler.

Within this report, organizations that provided information for the CSS report were revisited through websites to update figures given for 1988. If this was not possible, e-mails were sent directly to obtain an updated figure. In some instances, sources no longer held such information or simply did not reply; other organizations no longer existed.

From the number of sources provided in the CSS report, it can be assumed that a relatively small amount of data existed at that time. It follows from this that many of the figures presented in the report were based on assumptions and estimations by the authors. It was often the case that figures relating to the number of establishments (such as pet shops), employment and the revenue of such establishments were estimates, and figures were reported without confidence intervals and apparently accepted by the authors of the report. This poses challenges when trying to provide up-to-date figures.

The approach for updating figures began with broad Internet searches. Websites within the UK only were used. To establish the availability of data, broad terms were first used. Searches conducted were more to locate the sources that would hold the data, rather than assuming that data would be easily available. Terms and phrases such as '(UK) pet care industry' and 'pet care market' returned results for organizations associated with companion animals such as the Pet Food Manufacturers Association (PFMA), companion animal services, market research reports, and information on working in the animal care industry (Lantra). Searches were conducted in relation to specific factors, such as searching for the number and revenue of grooming establishments, and other companion animal services. A few attempts were made, changing words and phrases, to source data. If broader Internet searches were unsuccessful, further databases such as EBSCOhost and FAME (a database of companies) were used to source data and company financial information.

Charities, such as the Royal Society for the Prevention of Cruelty to Animals (RSPCA) and Dogs Trust, were known to produce and hold data on companion animals and were therefore consulted to aid the pursuit of data. Indeed, it became apparent early on through initial research that data were still quite limited, and that the data that did exist might be potentially unreliable. Therefore, greater use was made of charities; these were e-mailed, explaining the nature of the project and asking whether they held or knew of sources that could aid possible research. Replies received varied, with some unable to supply figures, whether due to resources or issues recording such data. In the event of information not being able to be sourced, or for any issues surrounding updating the information, comments have been provided in the relevant summary table (Appendix Table 1; www.cabi.org/openresources/91728) to highlight these issues and assist with the potential to gather better quality data in future. Appendix Tables 2 and 3 (www.cabi.org/openresources/91728) provide updated datasets.

UK economic data relating to companion animals and the associated industry has become of increasing value to many organizations, and a great quantity of data are found in market research reports. Websites of organizations such as Mintel, IBISWorld, Euromonitor and Datamonitor were visited, since they produce reports spanning many topic areas and they all have sections relating to various strands of the 'pet industry' in the UK and other geographical regions. Generally, the majority of reports related to pet food, pet accessories, pet insurance and veterinary services; excluding topics related to grooming and other companion animal services, suggesting that they are not of such considerable economic value. Of the large number of reports available, only three were used to provide illustrative examples of the data available, and the desire for the report to be largely based around

data that should be freely accessible to the public. These reports were analysed with economic data extracted and tabulated with notes made on the
trends in the market and reasons given for these changes. Interestingly, some
of the data given in the reports are from organizations such as the PFMA
and insurance companies, which are easily accessed through the Internet.

Technique for Data-mining Public Information

Where data relating to turnover, number of employees and the purpose of a
company were required, the FAME database was generally utilized. However,
annual reports for non-profit, voluntary organizations and charities associated with companion animals and assistance animals were specifically tar-
geted. Indeed, reports of this kind often contain valuable information and
data used to demonstrate their own economic and social value. Such reports
were obtained through organization websites, which were then analysed,
with figures and data being tabulated.

Reports were obtained from animal-related organizations and charities including: the RSPCA, People's Dispensary for Sick Animals (PDSA), Battersea,
Cats Protection, Dogs Trust, Wood Green, British Horse Society, The Donkey
Sanctuary and the Blue Cross. Factors were dependent on the organization's
report in question, but generally centred around: (i) stray, abandoned and
gifted animals; (ii) the number of volunteers and paid individuals working
for the organization; (iii) the economic value of volunteers' work; and (iv) the
revenue of the organizations. Other valuable data discovered and thought to
be potentially illuminating were also extracted and tabulated.

Reports from assistance-dog organizations included Guide Dogs for the
Blind, Hearing Dogs for Deaf People and Dogs for the Disabled (now Dogs
for Good), but were less readily available from some of the smaller charities,
though some data could be extracted from their websites. Figures extracted
and tabulated related to: (i) the current and past number of assistance-dog
partnerships created in the UK; (ii) the number of volunteers; (iii) costs associated with creating partnerships; and (iv) the revenue of the charities. Other
data thought to be of value have been extracted and tabulated.

Pet insurance companies such as NFU Mutual, Tesco, More Than,
Esure, Petplan, Churchill and Sainsbury's were approached to provide data
on a number of topics including: (i) obesity; (ii) common insurance holders'
claims; and (iii) the cost of companion animals (including food, accessories,
veterinary costs, services and insurance). The insurance company Petplan
had also produced a pet census for 2011. The websites of companies listed
were visited and explored for data. Data from such companies were reviewed, and in some cases figures presented were extracted and tabulated,
where they reflect the best data we could identify at the time.

Many topics associated with companion animals were found in the
public domain, through the press and public media. Journalists often

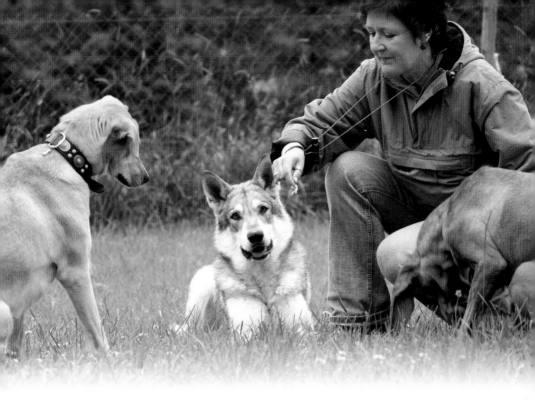

produce stories based on information obtained from academics, insurance companies, charities and other organizations. Media sites were not specifically visited and searched, but many articles were revealed from the Internet searches. Among the topics identified, subjects relating to companion animals and owners included: (i) exercise; (ii) the cost of owning companion animals; (iii) the price of pet insurance; and (iv) population statistics.

On finding a news article with data and figures of relevance, the figures or information were traced back to their original source. Where this could not be done, the figures were not used. For example, a series of press releases raised the issue of costs associated with police dog bites and animal rescues by fire services. These two topics were widely reported in many media outlets, yet the source was identified as being part of Radio 4 *You and Yours* documentaries, which in fact conducted its own investigative journalism and gained access to figures through sending the relevant freedom of information (FOI) requests. As the figures could be traced to a reliable source, they were extracted and tabulated (see Appendix Table 5; www.cabi.org/openresources/91728).

Health Literature

A wide literature now exists on the benefits of companion animals to their human owners, but this is of variable quality, and 'cherry picking' examples to make a case is always a danger. However, it is also important to recognize that similar studies that fail to find a significant effect do not refute the claims of these studies (absence of evidence is not evidence of absence), since they may be underpowered or reflect differences in content, such as population selection. They are, however, important cautions about over-generalization (Koivusilta & Ojanlatva, 2006). There is clearly a need for large multi-centric, international studies that might address these concerns. Until then each study needs to be carefully appraised as to its specific value. Several reviews have summarized potential human health benefits associated with companion animals (e.g. Serpell, 1990; McNicholas *et al.*, 2005; Barker & Wolen, 2008; Wells, 2009; McConnell *et al.*, 2011).

Illustrative findings from the literature include but are not limited to the following.

General health

- In a study that compared new pet owners to non-owners, those who acquired a pet experienced a highly significant reduction in minor health problems during the first month of pet ownership, and these benefits were sustained over time for dog owners. Dog owners also significantly increased their recreational walking, and this enhancement in physical activity was also maintained over time (Serpell, 1991).
- Having pets in the home has been linked to enhancements in general immune function in children, including reductions in respiratory infections, ear infections (Bergroth *et al.*, 2012) and gastroenteritis (Heyworth *et al.*, 2006).

Physical activity and healthy bodyweight management

- Regular physical activity improves mental health and reduces the risk of cardiovascular disease, hypertension, colon cancer, diabetes and a variety of other diseases (US Department of Health and Human Services, 1996). Dog owners appear to engage in more walking and physical activity than non-owners (Christian *et al.*, 2013) and are more likely to achieve recommended levels of physical activity (Coleman *et al.*, 2008; Cutt *et al.*, 2008; Oka & Shibata, 2009; Westgarth *et al.*, 2012).
- Older adult dog owners may be more than twice as likely to maintain their mobility over time as non-dog owners, and it is reported that they are more likely to walk faster and meet the recommended guidelines for physical activity (Thorpe *et al.*, 2006).

Cardiovascular health

- Pet owners may have a reduced risk of cardiovascular disease as they have significantly lower blood pressure, plasma triglycerides and cholesterol

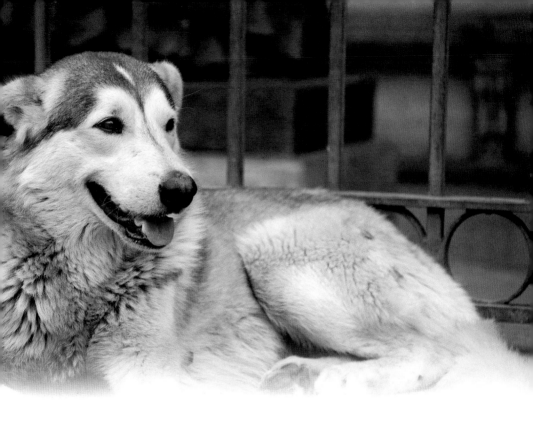

(Anderson *et al.*, 1992). Pet ownership has also been associated with improved 1-year survival rate for serious heart attacks. In this instance the evidence is considered strong enough for the American Heart Association to issue a statement in support of the role that pet ownership – particularly of dogs – can play in reducing the risk of developing cardiovascular disease (Levine *et al.*, 2013).

Allergies and asthma

- Childhood exposure to two or more dogs or cats has been reported to decrease the likelihood of developing certain kinds of allergic reactions later in life (Ownby *et al.*, 2002). Studies looking at the effects of exposure to pets in early childhood have found protective effects against the later development of both allergies and asthma (Hesselmar *et al.*, 1999; Platts-Mills *et al.*, 2001; Perzanowski *et al.*, 2002; Oberle *et al.*, 2003), but a recent study (Carlsen *et al.*, 2012) has highlighted the complexity of the issue, finding no association between furry and feathered animal keeping early in life and asthma in school age, but some evidence for an association between ownership during the first 2 years of life and a reduced likelihood of becoming sensitized to aero-allergens.

Mental health

- Children often seek out their pets when they are upset (Westgarth *et al.*, 2013) and view pets as confidantes and providers of support and comfort. Companion animals may also be ranked higher than certain human relationships in children's social networks (McNicholas & Collis, 2001). Social support can act as a buffer against the stresses of everyday life (Kikusui *et al.*, 2006) and it has been shown that people who share their homes with pets may have healthier physiological responses to stress, including lower baseline heart rate and blood pressure, and may demonstrate less cardiovascular reactivity to, and faster recovery from, mild stressors (Allen, 2001, 2003). The availability of social support has a profound effect on the physical and psychological well-being of people (Kikusui *et al.*, 2006) and non-pet owners have been reported to be twice as likely to frequently feel lonely than pet owners (Wood *et al.*, 2015).
- Cat owners have been reported to have fewer bad moods (Turner *et al.*, 2003) and have better psychological health than those who do not have pets (Straede & Gates, 1993). This may be, in part, because when cat owners are feeling depressed, they initiate more interaction with their cats, and the cats engage in more affectionate behaviour towards their depressed owners (Rieger & Turner, 1999). But clearly not every cat–owner relationship is a positive or mood-elevating experience (Ramos & Mills, 2009).
- Pets may ease the burden of bereavement particularly for those with relatively few confidants available (Garrity *et al.*, 1989; Adkins & Rajecki 1999). Pets may provide a buffer against the potential negative health consequences of bereavement, and a strong attachment to a pet has been associated with significantly less depression (Garrity *et al.*, 1989).

Studies that claimed to demonstrate that companion animals are of economic value were obtained, reviewed and evaluated. Many of the studies were obtained through searching scientific databases (e.g. Google Scholar™ scholarly texts search). The literature was themed into categories that presented a logical flow to demonstrate economic value (e.g. savings related to human health benefits). Specific searches were conducted to find further research relating to economic data, using EBSCOhost Online Research Database and Web of Science.

Assistance dogs have been included in their own category outside of their consideration under health and well-being, due to the wider economic impact of their work. Searches were conducted to identify the benefits of assistance animals through broad Internet searches and utilizing databases such as EBSCOhost. Reviews of existing studies were found, which gave detail of the benefits of assistance animals. In some

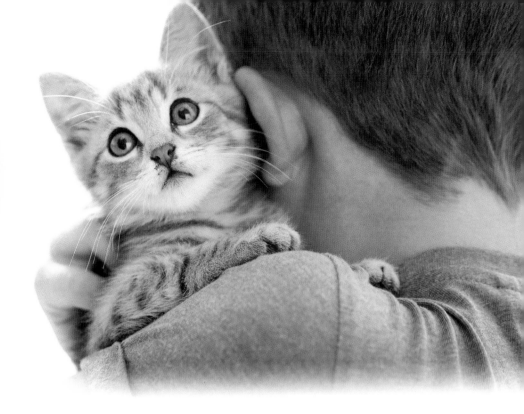

cases economic benefits were highlighted, such as reduced paid-assistance hours and increased employment.

Reliability of Information

The lack of reliable information in some areas poses challenges for this report, but overall the central message (i.e. that the economic significance of companion animals needs to be given serious academic consideration) is not diminished. This report is aimed at being a first step in raising awareness of the issues involved and their potential magnitude; it is hoped it will encourage the better recording and capture of data in future. Some figures evident through searches, and on websites such as www.petbusinessworld. co.uk, were excluded on the basis of being completely uncorroborated; however, given the lack of subsequent verifiable research, these figures may have proved useful to give some sort of indication of economic value.

The Yellow Pages™ is a source that has often been used in reports, including the CSS report. However, including figures from sources like the Yellow Pages™ within this current report was not a preferred method, as these were considered unreliable and often not a true representation of the number of establishments; not all establishments are listed, and searches in which terms differed slightly revealed conflicting figures. Using such sources was often a last resort, just to give an indication of the number of establishments within the UK. While pet shops, boarding establishments and some breeders require licenses to operate, the exact number of establishments could not be calculated even through sending FOI requests to all local authorities. Hence, this was not attempted but instead the deficit is noted within relevant tables.

The age of information was also important, as the most current figures were required. Indeed, in some instances data were dismissed on the basis of being outdated. An example of this was the imports and exports of tropical fish within the UK. The organization Ornamental Fish held some information on the number of fish traded and their economic value. However, the figures associated with this related to 1995. Not wanting to disregard these data totally, Ornamental Fish was contacted via telephone in order to see whether they maintained such figures. This communication revealed that they had tried to update the figures in collaboration with the Department for Environment, Food and Rural Affairs (Defra), but this had been unsuccessful. Existing data and figures were therefore excluded on the basis of being out of date.

Key Features of the Council for Science and Society (CSS) Report 1988

3

To put the current work in context, it is useful to review the scope and findings of the 1988 Council for Science and Society (CSS) report on animals in society, before considering the ways in which the figures may be updated, associated challenges and how the position of companion animals in society has developed (see later chapters). This was the first comprehensive evaluation of its kind to specifically consider companion animals in the UK. This report reflected on the extent and economic significance of the companion animal in society, as well as the benefits and problems that they bring.

The three main domains identified in the report were:

1. The extent and economic significance of the pet-keeping phenomenon.
2. The benefits of pet ownership.
3. The associated problems of pet ownership.

As we have noted already, the CSS report highlights the difficulty in distinguishing between the 'pet' and 'working' animal within some human–animal relationships. We retain the use of the term 'pet' in this chapter, in line with the original report.

Indicators of the Extent and Economic Significance of the Pet-keeping Phenomenon in 1988

Encompassing feeding, boarding and quarantine, accessories, grooming establishments and veterinary services, this section of the report provides an estimated total value of the companion animal-keeping phenomenon as a leisure activity amounting to £1.88 billion for dogs and cats alone, equivalent to about £4.6 billion in current money when adjusting for inflation (Retail Price Index in April 1988 was 105.8 and in April 2016 was 261).

© S. Hall, L. Dolling, K. Bristow, T. Fuller and D.S. Mills 2017. *Companion Animal Economics: The Economic Impact of Companion Animals in the UK* (S. Hall *et al.*)

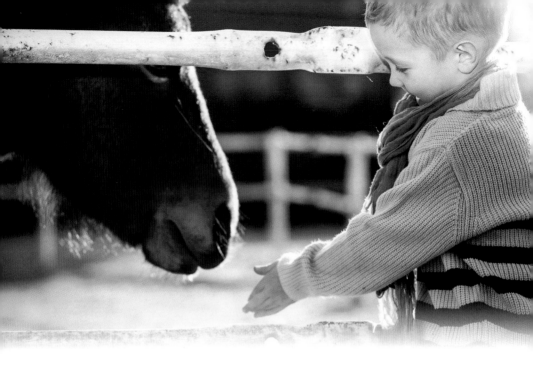

Perceived Benefits of 'Pet Ownership' in 1988

Benefits identified within the report include: (i) companion animals acting as a valuable educational experience for children (Levinson, 1972; Salmon & Salmon, 1983); (ii) the idea that dogs can act as 'social catalysts' to enhance social interaction within communities (Mugford & M'Comisky, 1975); (iii) studies indicating that dog ownership may help to increase the 1-year survival rate of heart attack patients (Friedmann *et al.*, 1980); (iv) the correlation between stroking companion animals and a reduction in heart rate and blood pressure (Katcher, 1981); (v) companion animals providing a source of recreation and exercise (Serpell, 1983); (vi) benefits in terms of offering a solution for loneliness and isolation, particularly for the older sector of the population (Bustad, 1980; Bustad & Hines, 1983); and (vii) more practical support offered by companion animals acting as deterrents towards burglars and intruders (Bennett & Wright, 1984).

As noted in the CSS report, the human–animal relationship potentially presents people with many desirable benefits, yet what is also apparent are the many variables to take into account. These include the nature of the perceived recipients of such benefits. Indeed, gender, age, circumstances and many equivalent features in the companion animal (as well as the species) all have the potential to be significant factors influencing what benefits are created. The quality of the relationship between owner and companion animal is also crucial in many instances and so it is an oversimplification to refer to the benefits of ownership as if these are the inevitable outcome of ownership. The American Veterinary Medical Association (AVMA) define the human–companion animal bond as 'a mutually beneficial and dynamic relationship between people and other animals that is influenced by behaviours that are essential to the health and well-being of both' (AVMA, 2006). The relationship that emerges is a dynamic phenomenon and there is clearly a need for better characterization of this, in order to make better predictions about who is likely to benefit and in what circumstances from companion animal ownership (see later discussion on passive versus active ownership).

Problems Associated with Pet Ownership in 1988

In order to provide a degree of balance, the associated problems of companion animal ownership and their impact on society as a whole are also considered in the 1988 report. We consider the specific costs of these in Chapter 4, but here we provide a brief summary of the key elements as it represents an important part of the initial report. Potential problems should not be overlooked, but the potential to mitigate against these in a way that does not undermine the value companion animals can provide should be given serious consideration. Simple bans are not an effective solution and are not an evidence-based solution (Orritt, 2014).

Companion animals can display problematic behaviours for their owners, such as undesirable reactivity in certain situations, destroying possessions or property, excessive noise, or other undesirable behaviours inside the home or out and about in the community as a result of a lack of training. Owners may also lack the resources or ability to effectively care for the animal, or perhaps become increasingly isolated from society as a result. These issues again raise concerns for the health and welfare of both the human and the animal, and are presented in the report as issues for both the animals themselves, as well as wider society. Problems with the abandonment and disposal of companion animals and the subsequent effect on shelters, charities and the animal itself are also considered within the 1988 report, alongside issues identified with the breeding and neutering of companion animals. In terms of the effect on the community, specific problems and the associated costs were calculated, to include canine pollution, disease and zoonoses, however, the costs associated with such diseases were not evaluated in monetary terms. Many of these issues are still relevant to society today, although there has been a marked reduction in public fouling by dogs following the introduction of the Dogs (Fouling of Land) Act 1996, which was subsequently replaced by the Clean Neighbourhoods and Environment Act 2005.

Estimates of the annual number of animal bites were also given, including dog attacks on delivery workers and the associated annual cost to the Post Office in sick pay. Figures for the annual number of road traffic accidents caused by dogs were also given within the 1988 report, and the burden of companion animals on farmers is also acknowledged, with the number of livestock killed annually and the subsequent compensation paid to farmers given.

Concluding Statements of the 1988 CSS Report

The CSS report was presented in the form of recommendations, a few of which centred around the need for further research into: (i) the manifestations and recognition of sentience in animals; (ii) the social, emotional and economic factors associated with abandonment, destruction and inadequate care of companion animals; and (iii) the potential psychological benefits of companion animals. Furthermore, recommendations included improvement in inspection of breeding premises, suggestions to minimize hereditary problems and cosmetic mutilations, proposal of a single

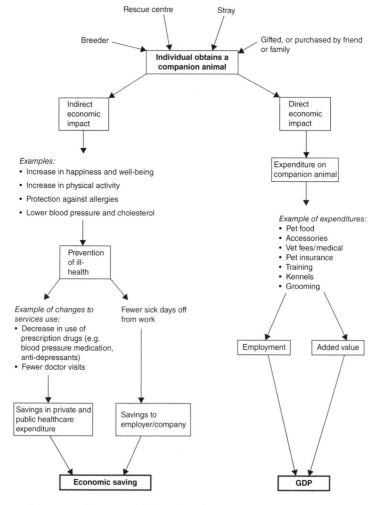

Fig. 3.1. Conceptual framework for identifying both direct and indirect economic benefits derived from companion animal ownership.

companion animal act, changes in the law relating to dogs on leads, improvement in exotic animal welfare, programmes of public education for companion animal owners, and support for a national dog licence. Many of these recommendations have still not been acted upon and remain important issues today.

The CSS report filled a niche at that time; it is an artefact of its time of publication. However, much of the data given in the CSS report was based largely on the assumptions and estimates of its knowledgeable authors. The birth of the Internet, since this time, has opened up the potential for greater data access on many of these important issues.

As the report highlights, further evaluation of the human–animal relationship is required to gain a fuller understanding as to the social, societal and individual benefits of companion animal ownership, and this is explored further in this report.

Unlike the CSS report, the current report aims to highlight the largely under-recognized economic value of companion animals to society, while acknowledging but not focusing on the problems that can arise from companion animals in society. To this end we propose here an initial conceptual framework to help appreciate from where potential economic benefits may derive (Fig. 3.1). A similar model could be applied to costs and it remains for future work to examine the full extent of these and the relative cost–benefit analysis of each.

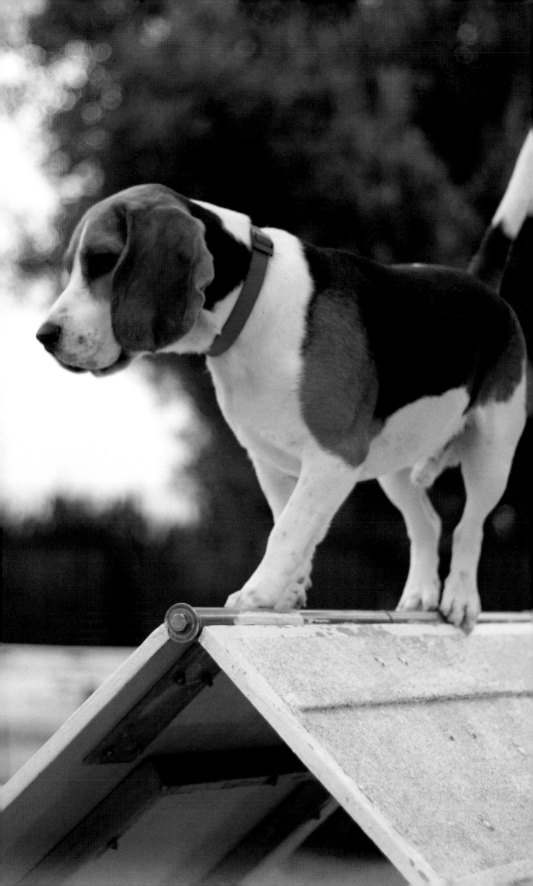

Updates on the Economic Impact of Companion Animals to the UK

4

Within the current report we make a number of references to the health benefits that companion animals may bring, and the associated potential economic savings related to this. However, it should also be documented that the scientific integrity on which these conclusions are based often fall below the traditional 'gold-standard' double-blind randomized control trial procedures. In general, human–animal interactions research is often criticized for using small sample sizes, a lack of random assignment to pet and no pet conditions, a lack of understanding or consideration of the causal relationship between health and pet ownership and the use of subjective, as opposed to objective, measures of assessment (O'Haire, 2010; Herzog, 2011). Nonetheless, even the authors who note these criticisms do not deny the potential for companion animals to benefit human health, and call for greater investment in research in this area. What does seem to be important is that researchers are encouraged to publish, and publicize, null-results relating to the impact of companion animals to health, as well as studies that report positive effects. Indeed, it is important that results are not 'cherry-picked' in favour of positive effects of companion animals in media reports and review articles.

One potential reason for disparity in this area is that research typically views ownership as a cohesive variable, whereas it is likely that companion animal ownership means different things to different people (e.g. depending upon their investment with their animal and their purpose for having the animal) and so the impact of companion animal ownership on different individuals is disparate. It is undoubtedly challenging to conduct controlled research in this area that matches up to the rigorous procedures applied to the single-intervention studies found in other areas of scientific enquiry, not least because a companion animal can often not be viewed as an 'independent variable'. Instead, the whole process associated with acquiring and living with a pet, together with the relationships that are formed, represents the intervention (Wright *et al.*, 2016). Traditional intervention studies in human health often

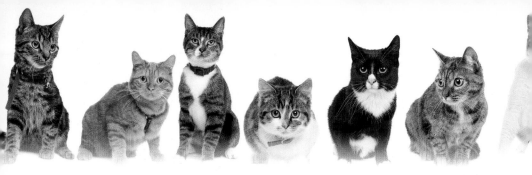

focus ideally on introducing a single variable (the treatment) in a blinded and placebo controlled way with participants randomly allocated to treatment and control groups. For many reasons it is difficult if not impossible to introduce some of these measures when studying the effects of companionship, not least because the relationship that develops is likely to be diverse (see earlier discussion on the problems of using 'ownership' as a metric, and later discussion on the difference between active and passive ownership). In animal intervention studies, the effect of the intervention probably extends from the relationship that is formed with the companion animal (and not the animal per se) and this will vary between subjects. Accordingly, it is possible that different subjects may accrue benefits through different mechanisms and the search for a singular mechanistic explanation may be an unrealistic scientific expectation. This failure to recognize the poor fit of companion animal-related interventions within traditional medical research paradigms may hinder wider recognition of their potential benefits among health professionals and academics alike (for an example of this see the discussion between Crossman & Kazdin, 2016, and Wright *et al.*, 2016). Furthermore, there is growing awareness in the applied and scientific health communities that interventions do not necessarily need, nor is it always relevant, to have control group comparisons to show a meaningful difference that has important implications for practice. For the purposes of this report, we are concerned with identifying potential impact, which if ignored could have a profound economic cost.

In order to present the current scope of the companion animal-keeping phenomenon and subsequent pet care industry, the 1988 indicators were sought so that they could be updated and extended. A discussion facilitating some of the issues and core themes discovered while conducting the research is presented here. In particular, we wish to draw attention to some of the possible benefits and costs to certain economies that are associated with companion animals.

Consideration of the Benefits and Costs of Companion Animals to the UK

The Council for Science and Society (CSS) (1988) report considered both benefits to the UK economy and some of the costs to the economy relating to the negative consequences of companion animals. We also believe it is necessary that, when evaluating the contribution of companion animals to the UK economy, both positive and negative aspects should be considered.

The CSS (1988) report discussed the implications surrounding animal abandonment, animal waste, diseases and accidents. We briefly consider how the figures in the CSS (1988) report have changed and what the implications of these figures are to the current economy.

Animal abandonment

The original CSS report indicated that, based on figures from the major dogs' homes, in large cities there may be around 300,000–400,000 dogs abandoned or lost a year and probably more than 50,000 cats, with a total 'surplus' of more than 500,000 a year. Updated figures indicate that around 50,000 dogs may be abandoned each year (*Vet Times*, 2015), and in 2014 Cats Protection alone rehomed more than 45,000 cats (Cats Protection, 2014) and the RSPCA reported rescuing more than 3000 cats (The Pet Site, 2014). This indicates that although the stray dog problem may have substantially declined, the cat problem has grown, which may partly reflect the increase in the number of cats owned. The average cost of caring for an abandoned cat is estimated at around £353, and double that amount for a dog (approximately £700) (Battersea, 2010). The total amount invested in caring for abandoned cats and dogs by Battersea in 2014 was £27,600 (Battersea, 2014). The CSS (1988) report indicated that urban shelters rehome around half their intake of abandoned animals, whereas rural shelters such as Wood Green Animal Shelter rehome 70–75% of cats and dogs and the National Canine Defence League (now Dogs Trust) rehomed about 80% of their dogs. Our updates show that Dogs Trust rehomed over 90% of their intake in 2015 (intake: 15,108; rehomed: 14,466) and Wood Green Animal Shelter rehomed over 70% of their intake (intake: 5720; rehomed: 4088). Although the costs of animal abandonment are not insignificant, they do also provide a source of employment for many UK residents. For instance, in 2014 Battersea employed 27 nurses, eight vets, three vet care assistants and a considerable number of kennel staff. Additionally, animal shelters are a point of interest to many families.

Urine

In 1988 it was reported that companion animals produced 4.5 million litres of urine and 1 million kg of faeces every day (1000 t/day). One of the major problems at that time was the lack of UK legislation to discourage dog fouling in public places, leading to hygiene hazards in streets, parks and playing fields. Although waste figures have risen considerably, estimated at around 3000 t/day, the introduction of legislation controlling fouling in public places (£50–80 fine; Gov.uk, 2016) has helped to reduce public hygiene concerns.

Diseases

Overall the number of reported zoonotic diseases relating to companion animals has declined since 1988, which may reflect increased hygiene standards and greater scientific advancements in healthcare. For instance, the number of cases of toxoplasmosis was 700 a year, but more recent figures indicate this has nearly halved to 325 a year in 2013 (see Appendix Table 2; www.cabi.org/openresources/91728). However, figures for *Pasteurella* infection have risen; between 1975 and 1984 there were 2937 cases (326 a year), and in 2013 there were 714 cases recorded (see Appendix Table 2; www.cabi.org/openresources/91728). Toxocariasis (a disease of humans caused by roundworm in the dog) is now considered a rare disease thanks largely to the development of better veterinary treatments and the control of fouling by dogs in public places. In total there are around 30 zoonotic diseases carried by dogs, including various forms of food poisoning, but some of these may also be transmitted from humans to dogs (anthroponeses). The role of companion animals in the rise of antibiotic-resistant infections is also a cause for concern, and although it is difficult to quantify, it should be given serious scientific attention (Guardabassi *et al.*, 2004).

Accidents

The number of reported bites from animals has also decreased. In 1988 the CSS reported around 99,000–200,000 bites/year from animals. Between 2013 and 2014 just over 7000 bites were reported from dogs and just over 3000 from other animals (2013–2014; see Appendix Table 2; www.cabi.org/openresources/91728). Similarly, numbers of attacks on delivery workers have also decreased, from 5560 in 1986 to 2976 in 2013–2014 (Royal Mail Group, 2012; Appendix Table 2; www.cabi.org/openresources/91728). In 2013, 1240 people living in the 10% most deprived areas were admitted to hospital for dog bites and 428 people living in the 10% least deprived areas were admitted (HSCIC, 2014). This combined total of hospital admissions for 20% of the country is 1668. The average cost of a non-elective inpatient hospital stay, excluding excess bed days, in 2013 was £1489 (Department of Health, 2013). Using these figures, the cost of hospital admissions due to animal bites in 2013 for 20% of the country was £2,483,652. This suggests that the often-quoted figure

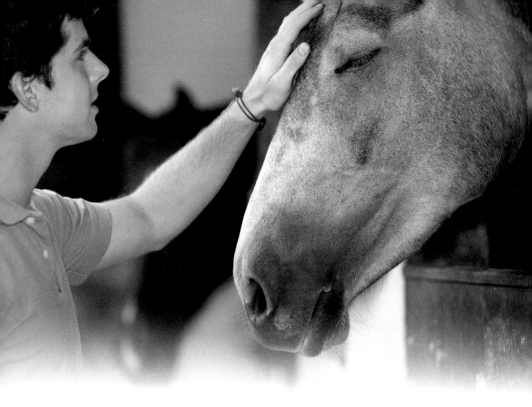

of around £3 million cost to the NHS from dog attacks (*The Telegraph*, 2014) may be a significant underestimate. If these averages are applied to the population, a figure of over £12 million is indicated. A conservative figure nearer £10 million may be more appropriate. Additionally, the legal costs surrounding dog bites and work days lost due to illness should be considered. However, it is challenging to obtain reliable figures relating to these issues.

Figures from the Royal Society for the Prevention of Accidents suggest that 75,000 dogs were involved in road accidents, resulting in 23 human fatalities (CSS, 1988). More recent data suggest a substantial decrease in these figures, with 32 serious road accidents involving a dog in 2004 and 254 slight accidents, resulting in one human fatality (see Appendix Table 2; www.cabi.org/openresources/91728). The Department for Transport no longer keeps data for the number of road traffic accidents involving dogs, therefore 2004 figures are the most current numbers available. Additionally, it is not possible to make a comparison with the number of livestock damaged due to companion animals as these records are no longer kept by the UK Government.

Companion Animal Population Statistics: Current Estimates

An important requirement of the current enquiry was to establish the size of the UK companion animal population, in the census period of 2011–2015. However, there is a lack of reliable, consistent figures relating to

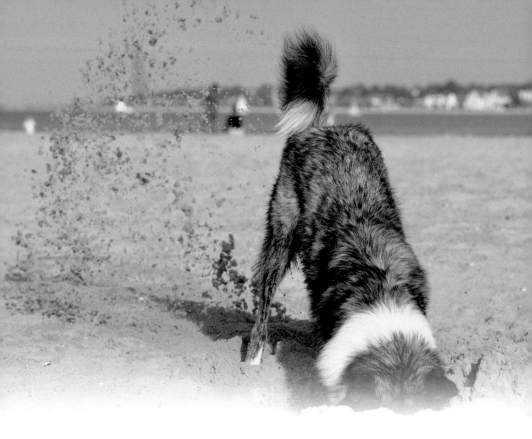

the number of animals within the UK. While such information is valuable to many sources including insurance companies, animal welfare charities, government officials, veterinary bodies and pet food manufacturers, no central database exists in the UK. One of the aims of this publication is to provide an initial focus for building such a database at the University of Lincoln.

In presenting the cat and dog population in 1988, the CSS report used information from the Pet Food Manufacturers Association (PFMA), representing 90% of the pet food manufacturing companies. For 2014, the PFMA estimated the cat and dog populations each at 'around 8–9 million'. For other species the approximated figures were: fish (45 million), rabbits (1 million), indoor birds (1 million), domestic fowl (1 million), guinea pigs (0.5 million), hamsters (0.5 million), horses and ponies (0.5 million) and tortoises/turtles (0.3 million). However, little information is provided about the methodology used to obtain such figures; only that a sample size of 6000 was surveyed. While these periodic population estimates are of use, the reliability of the figures is questionable. This is an important source of potential error when trying to upscale a prediction of the economic impact of one of these species at a national level.

Alternative figures based on a random sample of 2980 households in the UK, listed on the Register of Electors, have been produced (Murray

Table 4.1. Comparison of estimates of UK dog and cat populations provided by the Pet Food Manufacturers Association (PFMA) surveys and research based on random sampling from the electoral register (Murray *et al.*, 2010, 2015).

Type	PFMA estimation (2007)	Murray *et al.* estimation for 2006–2007[a]	PFMA estimations (2011)	Murray *et al.* estimation for 2011 ([+/-] 95% CI)[b]
Dog	7.3 million	10.5 million	8 million	11.60 (10.71–12.49) million
Cat	7.2 million	10.3 million	8 million	10.11 (9.14–11.04) million
Total	14.5 million	20.8 million	16 million	21.71 million

[a]Murray *et al.* (2010).
[b]Murray *et al.* (2015); CI, confidence interval.

et al., 2010). The data were collected in 2007 through telephone questionnaires. Two variables were used in order to predict the size of the population, which included the number of people in the household and the geographical location of the household (London/other areas of the UK). Other data used to predict figures consisted of 2001 UK Census data along with 2006 mid-year population estimates of the number of households and the average household size for England, Wales, Scotland and Northern Ireland. Their results suggested that the estimated size of the cat and dog population for 2006 was 10.5 million dogs and 10.3 million cats. In contrast to these figures, the PFMA for 2007 estimated the dog population at 7.3 million and the cat population at 7.2 million, indicating a potential underestimation of more than 30%. Murray *et al.* (2015) replicated the study on 2011 data, and estimated that there were around 12 million dogs and just over 10 million cats in the UK, whereas the PFMA data suggested figures of around 8 million for each, again indicating an underestimation of around 30%, even using the lower limits of their confidence intervals the underestimation is nearly 25% (Table 4.1).

It is acknowledged that the companion animal population is subject to fluctuation, but useful to note the percentage difference presented in the two estimates. If this is applied to the current estimates from PFMA, the combined dog and cat population could be more than 24 million for 2014, rather than the 17 million that they report.

Pet Food

As was the case in 1988, pet food and associated companion animal products are still reportedly the largest contributors to the pet care industry, with Mintel™ (2011) estimating the value of the market at £2.8 million. The PFMA (2014) reports that the value of the dog and cat food markets totalled £1.3 million and just over £1000 million, respectively. Furthermore, it has been noted that even through the economic downturn the pet food market has been maintained, which would suggest that companion animal owners are unwilling to compromise on what they feed their companion animals. Since 1988, the economic significance of this market appears to have been recognized by an increasing number of retailers, with a growth in the range of brands available, and many large supermarket chains now selling their own-brand products. Indeed, the cat and dog treat market alone is estimated to be worth £395 million/year (Pet Business World, 2016).

Most of the data surrounding the topic of pet food are readily available in market research reports. Interestingly much of the reasoning given in these reports for continued pet food market sustainability and expansion focused around words such as 'humanization' and 'anthropomorphism'. Indeed, it was widely commented that due to the increasing value placed on the lives of companion animals, owners have become increasingly conscious of what they feed to them. This has seemingly led to the expansion into specialist markets, such as organic food. Companies have been created solely on the premise of selling 'more natural' food for companion animals. For example, the ingredients listed by some companies refer to 'real' meat (whatever this may be), organic grains, organic vegetables and organic fruit and herbs, while excluding derivatives, colourings, flavourings, sweeteners or artificial preservatives.

Companion animal obesity has become an increasing concern within the UK, with various charities, organizations and companion animal companies raising awareness of the issue. Overweight pets are reported to be one of the top concerns of small animal vets (PFMA, 2014), these animals are subject to a range of additional health risks associated with this problem such as cancers, skin diseases, high blood pressure, heart disease, diabetes mellitus, orthopaedic disease and respiratory distress. However, the rising awareness of obesity and associated health issues has provided further opportunities for the pet food industry in the form of weight reduction food for animals to help support weight loss programmes.

The 'Pet Shop': the Evolution of Allied Industries in the Companion Animal Care Sector

While in 1988 a simple estimation could be given for the number of pet shops that existed, to do so now would be more complicated. As the roles of companion animals have evolved within society, so have the outlets at which companion animal owners purchase pet food, accessories and products.

Since the CSS report, as with the trend in food retailing for humans, there has been a general decline in independent pet shops and an increase in larger 'pet supermarket' chains such as Pets at Home, Jolleyes, Pets Corner,

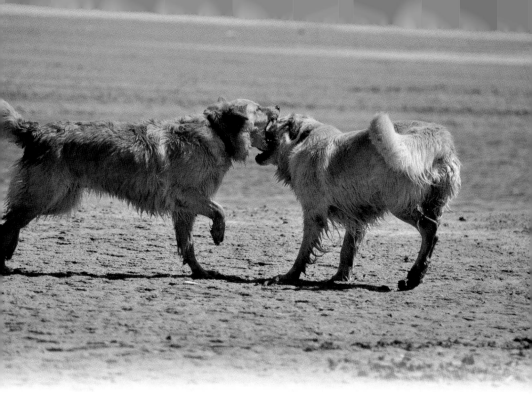

Just for Pets and Partners Pet Supermarket, alongside an increased presence in normal supermarkets such as Tesco, Asda, Morrisons and Sainsbury's.

Pets at Home, established just 2 years after the publication of the CSS report, is by far the largest of the pet supermarkets. They sell a wide range of products and services, from feed to novelty products, veterinary centres, grooming salons and hydrotherapy. At the time of our initial census in 2011, the chain consisted of 287 stores nationwide, employed 3092 individuals, and had an annual turnover of £468 million. Updates on figures since this time show that by summer 2014, over 350 stores were operating, with over 5000 staff employed and an estimated value of £1 billion and revenue of £665.4 million (see Appendix Table 3; www.cabi.org/openresources/91728). This dramatic increase in figures provides a brief illustration of the strength of the pet market in today's society.

More recently, there has been a rise in online specialist retailers such as Petmeds.co.uk, Zooplus.co.uk, PetLifeOnline.co.uk, PetPlanet.co.uk and Pet-Supermarket.co.uk. Such retailers sell a range of products, including pet food, health products and accessories, over the Internet, enabling owners to shop in comfort and at their own convenience. Taking PetPlanet.co.uk as an example, in 2010 they had on offer 10,470 products to 813,594 registered online members, and had an annual turnover of around £6.5 million (see Appendix Table 3; www.cabi.org/openresources/91728), a figure that doubled in the 5 years since the initial census undertaken for the current report.

The creation of such specialist pet stores could indicate that companion animals have become of increasing importance within human lives, and their rapid growth poses challenges to estimating their current economic impact. Thus many of the figures given here should be considered illustrative for raising awareness of the economic significance of companion animals, rather than absolute fact.

Companion Animal-related Services: Shifting Dynamics of Services

Companion animal services were not commonly found to be the focus of reports, which may be because such services are often run on a small scale and by independent businesses, but it seems clear that this area has grown since the CSS report. Although not representing a dramatic increase, expansion into services such as mobile grooming, 'pet sitting', dog walking and training, companion animal taxis and the management of the death, memorial or disposal of companion animals has evolved over time. This may relate to the importance of the relationships that develop through companionship, since many owners now seek to provide 'a dignified end and farewell' for their loved ones. This has led to a rise in the number of pet funeral services, individual pet cremations and pet cemeteries. Some owners also explore taxidermy services and cloning the deceased is now a reality. For those that do have trouble coming to terms with the loss of a companion animal, bereavement services, such as the Animal Samaritans and Pet Bereavement Support Service from the Blue Cross Charity, provide understanding and support for grieving owners.

Although many pet services are small-scale independent establishments, they still have a large impact economically. According to Lantra (2010), the companion animal care industry employs 78,000 people in 12,650 businesses. It would appear that there is an increasing need and desire for companion animal services, which is subsequently supporting diverse lines of small business employment.

Companion Animal Health: Parallels with Human Health

Since 1988, there has been a significant increase in the advancement of veterinary healthcare for animals. Over time, companion animals have become of increasing personal importance to their owners, with a greater emphasis placed on improved healthcare. The turnover of the veterinary market within

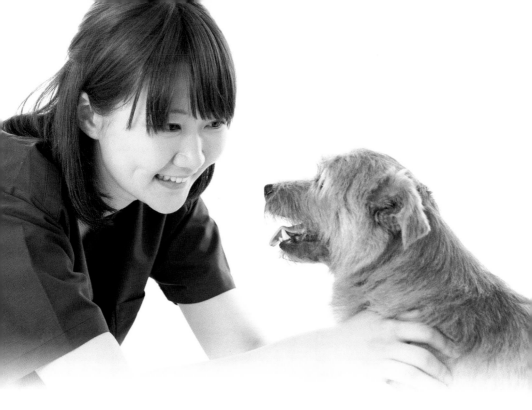

the UK in 2015 is estimated at £3 billion, with 3621 businesses, and 51,411 people employed (IBIS World, 2011). The technology within these businesses has also expanded and created new opportunities for service providers here as well. The number of recognized animal hospitals has increased since 1988 and this represents substantial economic investment in the sector, with some of these hospitals equipped with MRI and CT scanners, hydrotherapy pools and various other state-of-the art medical facilities that might be found in a human hospital. For example, Glasgow University's relatively new Small Animal Hospital cost an estimated £15 million when opened in 2009.

The apparent increased value placed on the lives of companion animals has corresponded with a greater economic value of veterinary services; and an increase in companion animal insurance since 1988. Total paid claims in 2014 amounted to more than £600 million, or £1.65 million/day (Association of British Insurers, 2015).

Companion animal insurance is now offered through numerous outlets including traditional insurance companies, supermarkets and charities. Some of these companies do not sell products related to companion animals other than insurance. While the increase in companion animal insurance seemingly allows owners to afford treatment for their companion animals, this has also had an impact on the associated annual cost of owning a companion animal. Data relating to the increasing annual cost of companion

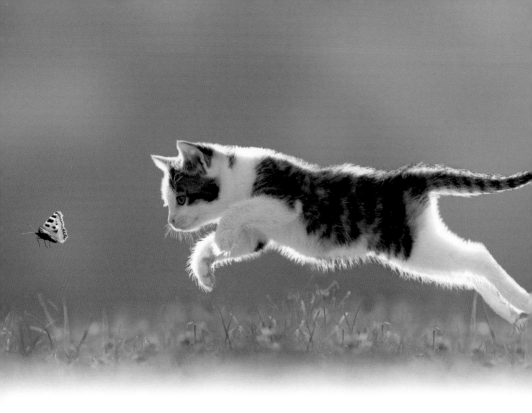

animals is a frequently discussed topic within the media, with many contra-
dictory annual estimates being given. It is worth noting that a recent report
suggests that the lifetime cost of a healthy dog may be between £16,000 and
£31,000, and a cat around £17,000 (Statista, 2015) (i.e. these are the costs
including general care and preventive treatments but excluding veterinary
medical treatment).

Indirect Costs: Extending the Scope of Economic Value

The previous chapter considered direct economic costs, however, there is growing recognition that companion animals also provide many significant indirect financial benefits (still referred to as costs in economic terms). In this chapter, two areas are chosen to illustrate the significance of indirect costs associated with companion animals: (i) the effect of companion animal ownership on human health (considering examples relating to the physical, mental and social health of people) and its economic implications; and (ii) the additional health benefits of economic value provided by animal-assisted interventions and the wider support of individuals with increased need in our society. Other pet-assisted activities are likely to provide indirect economic benefits (e.g. Pets as Therapy (PAT) dogs, the Kennel Club's Bark and Read programme) but no evaluative data could be sourced.

5A HUMAN HEALTH AND WELL-BEING

As predicted in the CSS report (1988), recognition of the perceived benefits for human health and well-being associated with companion animals has continued to grow since the small number of studies reported at that time. However, the quality of the studies is variable and does not always support some of the claims made; thus the perceived benefits should be approached with caution (see earlier discussion).

Since 1988, there has been much research indicating that interactions with dogs can provide emotional and physical health benefits for diverse human populations: bringing together communities (Zimolag & Krupa, 2009; Wood *et al.*, 2015), serving as facilitators of social communication (Esteves & Stokes, 2008), lowering levels of anxiety (Barker *et al.*, 2010), providing opportunities to share experiences and learn new skills (Gee *et al.*, 2009) and to engage with the natural world (Pederson *et al.*, 2012). They clearly have an important preventive health role through shaping human

© S. Hall, L. Dolling, K. Bristow, T. Fuller and D.S. Mills 2017. *Companion Animal Economics: The Economic Impact of Companion Animals in the UK* (S. Hall et al.)

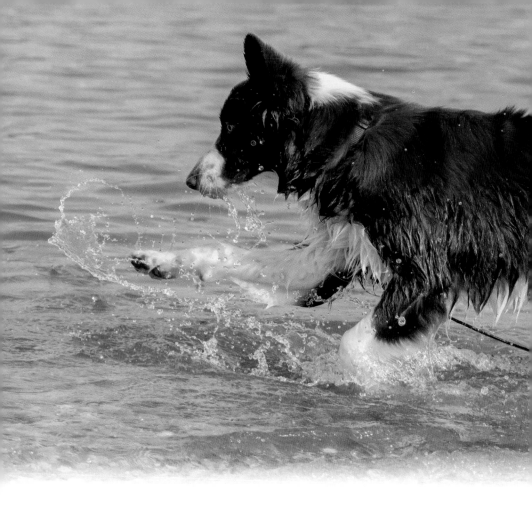

emotional and cognitive development more generally (Mills & Hall, 2014). Such studies lead us to consider the wider economic implications of perceived benefits on the healthcare system, thus potentially generating economic savings.

Recovery from Major Illness

There is a growing body of literature suggesting that owning a dog can potentially aid recovery from major illness or surgery. Still one of the most widely cited studies in support of the benefits of companion animals to those with major illness is that of Friedmann *et al.* (1980). This study suggested that companion animal ownership, particularly dog ownership, is associated with a higher 1-year survival rate following coronary heart disease, in comparison to non-owners. Such results suggest that having a companion animal may decrease heart attack mortality by 3%, thus saving around 30,000 lives annually. While this early study received criticism relating to methodological weakness (Wright & Moore, 1982), it has since been replicated (Friedmann & Thomas, 1995), extending the number of participants, and again concluded that those participants who owned a dog were more likely to be alive 1 year after a heart attack than those who did not. The range of major illnesses examined in this context has also been extended, for example one study indicates that owning a dog was associated with significantly better perceived control of illness and treatment for women who have breast cancer (McNicholas *et al.*, 2001).

While both studies present associations between companion animal ownership and enhanced survival rates, the studies themselves do not address the role of the companion animals in recovery, nor do they provide a specific mechanistic basis for these effects. The studies postulate that outcomes could be mediated through the act of stroking a companion animal, causing a calming effect and consequently lowering heart rate.

Prevention of Ill-health

As well as reportedly aiding recovery, companion animal owners are also perceived to have better general health than non-owners. Many studies focus on the relationship between companion animal ownership and the associated benefits to cardiovascular health including decreasing the blood pressure of the owner (Anderson *et al.*, 1992; Allen, 2001) and reduced risk of heart attack (Qureshi *et al.*, 2009). Studies suggest that short-term decreases in blood pressure and heart rate may occur through the acts of talking to or stroking a dog (Katcher *et al.*, 1983; Baun *et al.*, 1984; Vormbrock & Grossberg, 1988). Just being in the presence of a dog is reportedly associated with a decrease in blood pressure (Friedmann *et al.*, 2007). It has also been suggested that blood pressure levels were significantly lower for individuals that had a positive attitude towards dogs, in contrast to those with a more negative attitude (Friedmann & Lockwood, 1993). Indeed, the evidence in favour of the positive value of companion animals in relation to cardiovascular disease has now reached a level of strength to be formally recognized by the American Heart Association (Levine *et al.*, 2013).

Children are also reported to have health benefits from companion animal ownership. It is suggested that exposing typically developing children to companion animals during the first year of life might be associated with a lower frequency of allergic rhinitis, asthma and eczema (Hesselmar *et al.*, 1999; Karimi *et al.*, 2011; Davis & Belnap, 2013), but the effect may vary with the number of animals in the home (Ownby *et al.*, 2002). A recent systematic review of the subject highlights the complexity of the issue, by concluding dogs in particular may reduce the risk in families without a history of asthma, but increase risk in high-risk groups (Lodge *et al.*, 2011). Further research is justified and simple generalizations should be guarded against.

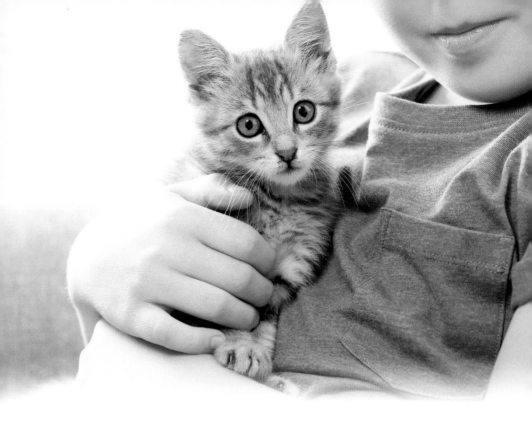

An important British study by Serpell (1990) reported that individuals who had recently acquired a dog or cat reported a highly significant reduction in minor health problems (such as coughs, dizziness and hay fever) as well as a dramatic increase in the number and duration of recreational walks. However, the World Health Organization defines health as 'a state of complete physical, mental and social well-being and not merely the absence of disease or infirmity' (World Health Organization, 1946); and so the potential impact of companion animal ownership on each of these aspects of well-being needs to be considered, since each may be associated with indirect economic costs of value to society.

Physical Well-being: Passive versus Active Ownership – Enhanced Physical Exercise

The considerable literature relating to the effects of dog ownership on physical activity has recently been brought together in a review (Christian *et al.*, 2013). The review highlights an important feature relating to the impact of companion animals on human health, which we term passive and active ownership. Passive ownership refers to the incidental effects accruing from ownership that depend on the presence of the animal in the home (e.g. potential effects on the risk of asthma discussed above), whereas active ownership refers to the effects from the lifestyle adopted when owning a companion animal. The latter are less reliably associated with 'ownership' per se since they are dependent on other factors that are enabled (but not enforced) by ownership. This might include the tendency to be more active.

Several studies indicate that dog ownership is associated with greater physical activity and recreational walking for owners (see Christian *et al.*, 2013 for a review), which has the potential and ability to produce health benefits for the individuals (e.g. Ham & Epping, 2006; Cutt, 2007). Dog walkers themselves have demonstrated that although not always wanting to go outside and walk, motivation for doing so was often attributed to the presence of the dog (Knight & Edwards, 2008).

Again, it is suggested that children also benefit, with claims that children from dog-owning families spend more time in light or moderate to vigorous activity, in comparison to children without dogs (Salmon, 2007; Owen *et al.*, 2010; Salmon *et al.*, 2010). Further research by Timperio *et al.* (2008) observed that the odds of being obese or overweight were lower among children aged 5–6 years (but not significant for ages 10–12 years). These data were adjusted for school, sex, physical activity, parental weight, maternal education and neighbourhood; accordingly, owning a dog could protect children in this age range from being overweight.

However, in many cases the link with perceived health benefits may lie elsewhere since not all dog owners walk their dogs (Oka & Shibata, 2009).

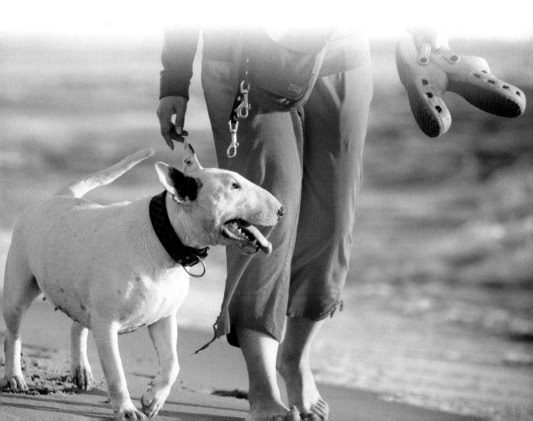

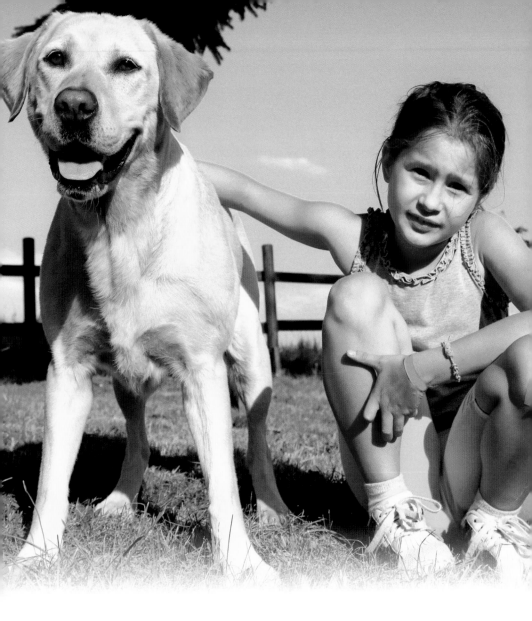

Indeed, an Australian study (Bauman *et al.*, 2001) revealed that more than half of dog owners did not walk their dogs, and were less likely to meet recommended levels of activity sufficient for health benefits. The authors observed that if all dog owners were to walk their dogs for 30 minutes each day, this could lead to substantial disease prevention and potential health-care cost savings of AUS$175 million/year; so perhaps there is value in promoting responsible pet ownership and the need to 'walk the dog' for more than the dog's benefit. As well as enhancing physical activity, dog walking has also been shown to result in significantly higher numbers of chance conversations with complete strangers than walking without a companion animal (McNicholas & Collis, 2000), and this may improve social well-being.

Social Well-being: Enhanced Social Contacts/Interactions

An increase in frequency of social interactions has been reported not only when out walking the dog but also when engaged in a range of normal daily activities where the dog could be included. Furthermore, it is suggested that owning a dog contributes to a far greater extent to the building of social networks (Upton, 2005) and in some cases dogs can facilitate relationships that are more than just conversational interactions (Guéguen & Ciccotti, 2008). The indirect impact of the improved health associated with this type of interaction does not appear to have been modelled from an economic costs perspective.

Mental Well-being: Elevating Mood and Increasing Mental Resilience

Alongside facilitating greater social interaction, companion animals have also been shown to reduce loneliness in certain sectors of the population. For example, women that were living alone have been reported as being significantly lonelier than those living with companion animals, suggesting that companion animals can diminish the feelings of loneliness and isolation (Zasloff & Kidd, 1994). A study on bonds between the elderly and their dogs (Peretti, 1990) suggested that many individuals believed their dog to be their only friend and one that could match a human bond, therefore being able to fulfil their owners' psychological needs for attachment and nurturance. However, a Canadian study by Antonacopoulos and Pychyl (2010) found that dog owners and non-dog owners with low levels of human support did not report a difference in loneliness, yet among those groups with high levels of human support, dog owners were shown to be significantly less lonely than non-owners.

It is widely believed that owning a companion animal may also prevent and alleviate symptoms of mild depression, and therefore reduce the risk of a wide range of other problems with related economic costs. Indeed, merely owning a companion animal can serve to provide individuals with structure and routine, thereby giving individuals a feeling of purpose and self-esteem. Studies have also indicated that individuals owning companion animals have better psychological well-being (Serpell, 1990; Straede & Gates, 1993; Bennet *et al.*, 2015), with companion animal owners reporting greater happiness and health compared with non-owners (McConnell *et al.*, 2011).

A common theme in animal-companionship literature is the anxiety-(which has a strong co-occurrence with depression) reducing effects that animals have in a range of individuals (Lang *et al.*, 2010; Berget & Grepperud, 2011; Dietz *et al.*, 2012). In 2007, 2.28 million people in the UK were diagnosed with an anxiety disorder, which cost the economy approximately £8.9 billion. It is projected that by 2026, 2.56 million anxiety-related diagnoses will be made, which will cost the economy approximately £14.2 billion (McCrone *et al.*, 2008). Just over half the people living with an anxiety disorder do not receive treatment, which is associated with lost employment costs. However, if 95% of people with anxiety disorders were to receive treatment, service costs would double (from £1.2 billion to approximately £2.1 billion; McCrone *et al.*, 2008). The ability of companion animals to prevent and remediate symptoms of anxiety independent of medical services is exciting and worthy of further controlled investigations.

Families are also shown to benefit through the acquisition of a companion animal, with increases in family happiness and fun being reported (Cain, 1985). Mechanistic explanations for an increase in well-being have been proposed in some studies. For instance, Odendaal (2000) demonstrated that simply interacting with a dog has the ability to decrease levels of stress and enhance levels of dopamine and endorphins associated with happiness. Furthermore, active and passive interaction with a companion animal have also been shown to reduce levels of anxiety, and reduce the onset, severity or progression of stress-related conditions in certain circumstances (Wilson, 1991). Therefore, it has been suggested that dogs can be a preventive and therapeutic measure against everyday stress (Allen *et al.*, 1991). Recent research on families with an autistic child indicate that a family dog may be particularly important for the carers of such children (Wright *et al.*, 2015b).

Companion animals have also been identified as potentially aiding owners and family adolescents (Siegel, 1995; Black, 2012) through stressful life events (Mills & Hall, 2014). Indeed, people are often susceptible to becoming depressed during such times, yet owning a companion animal may help, possibly even to the point of reducing the need for older companion animal owners to enter the healthcare system (Siegel, 1990; Raina *et al.*, 1998).

Some studies have focused on the role companion animals can have in particular life-changing events. For example, patients with AIDS reported that their companion animals provided support, companionship and a purpose, thereby reducing feelings of loneliness and depression compared with those patients who did not own companion animals (Carmack, 1991; Siegel *et al.*, 1999; Castelli *et al.*, 2001). Companion animals have also been reported to help women recovering from breast cancer, possibly through providing valuable emotional and tactile support (McNicholas *et al.*, 2001).

Loss of a loved one can also potentially lead to depression, yet individuals currently coping with the loss of a loved one have been reported to show fewer symptoms of physical and psychological disease than in those individuals that did not own companion animals (Akiyama *et al.*, 1987).

A common theme emerging from the studies above is that during times of change, or when exposed to events that can place individuals at a higher risk of conditions like depression, companion animals appear to be able to play a significant role in increasing the resilience of the owner. This might result in fewer visits to the doctor and be of significant economic value; this cost has been modelled in other countries, as we discuss in the next section.

Fewer Visits to the Doctor

Many of the studies already presented imply cost savings through such notions as preventing ill health and aiding survival. However, discussions around economic impact in relation to human health appear to be focused primarily on companion animal ownership resulting in fewer doctor visits. Several studies have been conducted in countries such as the USA, Australia, Germany and China, but few in the UK (Philips, 2002, cited in Fine, 2010).

Headey (1995) observed that Australian companion animal owners, from various demographics, made fewer doctor visits than non-owners. Furthermore, the same companion animal owners were also reportedly less likely to be taking medication for heart problems, high blood pressure, high cholesterol and sleeping difficulties. Such observations of fewer doctor visits and decreased medication use present the possibility of health cost savings. It was also noted that certain sectors of the population associated with higher use of the healthcare system (young women, older women and older men) were the greatest beneficiaries of companion animal ownership. However, as with many such studies, the mechanism whereby companion animal ownership might cause such desirable outcomes is unknown. It was hypothesized that companion animal ownership may improve health through encouraging owners to take more exercise (such as walks) and by improving social networks and/or reducing loneliness, leading to a reduction in medication taken and fewer doctor visits (see Fig. 5.1), but other mechanisms may well be involved as well.

Headey and Grabka (2007) conducted a further robust longitudinal study of the German and Australian population. They showed that people

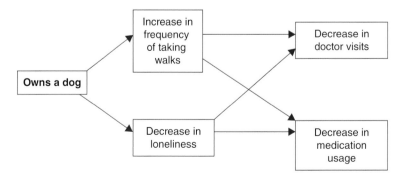

Fig. 5.1. Hypothesized mechanisms as to why companion animal ownership may lead to fewer visits to the doctor. (From Headey, 1995.)

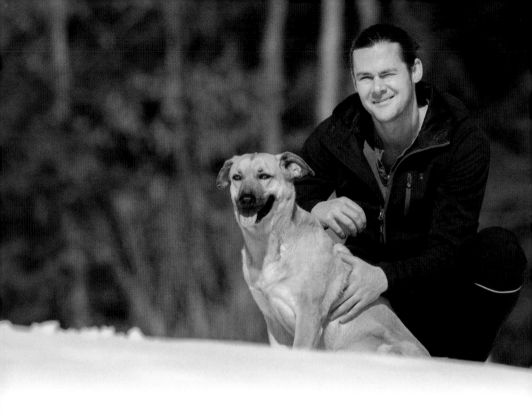

who own a companion animal are healthier than those who ceased to have one or never had one. It was shown that companion animal owners make 15% fewer annual visits to their doctors than non-owners. Furthermore, research conducted in China, where companion animals were banned until 1992, revealed that dog-owning women aged 25–40 years self-reported greater exercise per week, greater fitness and health, fewer bad nights' sleep, fewer days off sick from work and fewer doctor visits, in comparison with those not owning a dog (Headey *et al.*, 2008).

Given the ageing population both nationally and globally, the significance of this effect may be of increasing importance to both governments and healthcare providers. There are good data to support that the effect extends to seniors (Siegel 1990; Raina *et al.*, 1998). Stressful life events appear to be associated with increased doctor visits for individuals without companion animals, and thus companion animals, particularly dogs, seemingly help families in stressful times by acting as 'stress buffers', reducing respondents' need to enter the healthcare system. Raina *et al.* (1998) reported that among non-institutionalized seniors, companion animal owners had a mean of 30 encounters with the healthcare system in comparison to 37 for non-companion animal owners. Therefore the average cost of companion animal owners (US$530) was lower than that of non-companion animal owners (US$694). The results of this study are, however, somewhat confounded by the admission that companion animal owners were more likely to be married or living with someone, younger, and more physically active that non-companion animal owners, suggesting that other variables may also have had an impact on the perceived outcomes. Nonetheless, given the potential significance of this, it deserves further investigation. Until now, little attempt has been made to cost the likely significance of this factor to the UK economy, but we describe and undertake the exercise in the next section.

Economic Impact: A Preliminary Estimation

A recent report in the USA suggested that, as a conservative estimate, companion animal ownership may save healthcare services around US$12,000 million a year (Clower & Neaves, 2015). However, this figure has been challenged on the basis that the evidence of benefit is not as clear as claimed; there is confusion between correlation and causality when it comes to assessing the effects of companion animals on human health, and finally there are healthcare costs to keeping a pet, such as the cost of animal injuries (Herzog, 2016). These criticisms have merit, but they do not mean that the potential benefits should be dismissed out of hand; rather it is important for policy makers to take note of all evidence and consider whether further investigation is warranted. When trying to make real-life decisions about complicated issues, an important question that needs to be addressed is: what are the costs of being wrong? In this context, the evidence indicates that the economic benefits of companion animals deserve consideration, and the assumptions need to be clearly stated.

Clearly the issue is complicated. If we take the example from the previous section, the authors make plausible linkages, illustrated in Fig. 5.2. There are many variables to be taken into account, and a number of factors that can impact such outcomes. Specific testing of the various hypotheses is possible if funding is forthcoming, but the absence of this does not negate

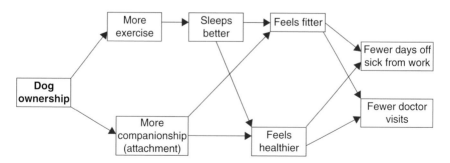

Fig. 5.2. Hypothesized potential mechanisms as to why companion animal ownership may lead to fewer days off sick from work and fewer visits to the doctor. (From Headey et al., 2008.)

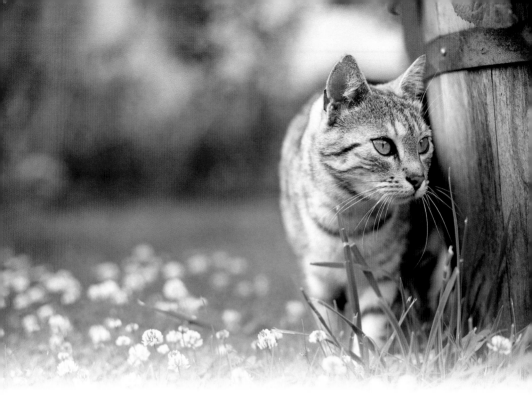

the observation that there are many potential variables relating to fewer sick days and doctor visits to suggest potential economic savings.

At this point it is worth considering one of the pioneering studies in the estimation of the economic savings associated with companion animal ownership and its context. Headey and Anderson (1995) originally attempted a preliminary estimate of the possible government and public healthcare expenditure savings in Australia, due to the apparent links between companion animal ownership and better health. Estimates were based on data obtained from the 1994 Australian National People and Pets Survey, which indicated, among other things, that fewer doctor visits are associated with companion animal owners compared with non-companion animal owners. The study was conducted on the basis of comparing actual Australian health expenditure for 1992/93 (AUS$32,922 million) with a counterfactual situation where companion animals did not exist or were banned. It was observed that the difference between current expenditure and the hypothetical expenditure in the absence of companion animals can be regarded as the savings due to companion animals.

As visits to general practitioners (GPs) are generally the first point of contact with the healthcare system for many, it was assumed that healthcare expenditure can be apportioned on the basis of doctor visits. Another consideration taken into account is the people who receive health benefits from companion animal ownership. It is assumed that as well as main carers receiving benefits, other family members will benefit to half the extent. It was estimated that healthcare savings for main carers was AUS$790 million. Savings for additional family members, receiving benefits to half the extent of the main carer, was estimated at AUS$749 million, giving a total overall savings of AUS$1539 million in healthcare expenditure. A more conservative, yet less realistic, method was also given, estimating the savings for main carers at AUS$262 million. This estimate was produced through directly calculating: (i) savings from fewer GP visits by companion animal owners; (ii) savings due to lower consumption of pharmaceuticals; and (iii) savings due to assumed lower rates of hospitalization among companion animal owners.

Headey (1998) later revised the figures using health expenditure in Australia for 1994/95 (AUS$36.591 billion). A saving of AUS$988 million, equivalent to 2.7% of the nation's health expenditure, was reported. In addition to this, another AUS$825 million was calculated for health benefits towards family members, thus producing an overall estimated cost saving of AUS$1813 million (5% of the total health expenditure).

Possible Contribution to UK Healthcare Expenditure Savings

The above methods used to calculate the savings to the Australian economy can be used to replicate the potential savings for UK healthcare expenditure, given similar assumptions. Data used in the calculation are those for 2013 except where indicated. The steps used to calculate the possible healthcare expenditure savings are the same as presented in Headey (1998). The primary assumption is that visits to the doctor can be used as a proxy for total healthcare usage and thus expenditure on different populations. The steps are as follows.

Step 1: UK healthcare expenditure

In 2013, UK healthcare expenditure came to a total of £124 billion, 8% of GDP (gross domestic product) (UK Public Spending, 2013).

Step 2: Population estimates

In 2013, 63.5 million people lived in the UK in 26.4 million households (ONS, 2013), with 46% owning a cat and/or a dog (Murray *et al.*, 2015). This indicates that there are around 12.14 million main companion animal carers ('owners', assuming one per household) who may be in better health than those non-companion animal owners. Owners therefore formed 19.1% of the population in 2013. The remaining 80.9% of the population were not primary companion animal owners, and while some will live in households with companion animals, for the purposes of this calculation

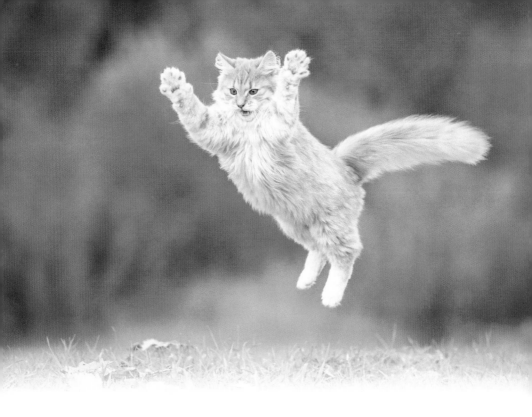

we will assume they do not to receive any health benefits due to companion animals (despite evidence to the contrary that family members may receive benefit at a level of 50%; however, this assumption helps make our calculation a conservative estimate).

Step 3: Doctor visits

In 2008 it was estimated that the average person makes 5.5 visits to their GP each year (Hippisley-Cox & Vinogradova, 2009).

Headey and Grabka (2007) estimated that in Australia, companion animal ownership reduced the number of GP visits by around 11%, whereas in Germany the effect size was around 24%. For the purpose of this study, in order to be conservative, we will estimate a 10% reduction. Accordingly:

$$0.191(x) + 0.809(y) = 5.5; \; x = 0.9y$$

where y is the number of visits made to the GP by a non-animal owner (80.9% of population) and x the number of visits made to the GP by an animal owner (19.1%). This gives us a figure of 5.61 for y, and a value of 5.04 for companion animal owners (90%y).

Based on the figures represented in Table 5.1, it is estimated that the 80.9% of the population who did not own a cat or dog made 82.5% of annual doctor visits. Although the total estimate for doctor visits exceeds that calculated

Table 5.1. Visits to the doctor by cat and dog owners versus non-owners.

Proportion of population	Doctor visits per year	Total doctor visits (million)	Total doctor visits (%)
Dog and cat owners (19.1% = 12.14 million)	5.04	61.19	17.5
All others (80.9% = 51.36 million)	5.61	288.13	82.5
Total	5.5[a]	349.32	100

[a]In 2008 it was estimated that the average person makes 5.5 visits to the doctor each year (Hippisley-Cox & Vinogradova, 2009).

for the year (Hippisley-Cox & Vinogradova, 2009), this probably relates to unregistered patients and we have no way of knowing whether these are more or less likely to be pet owners. Thus we have assumed that the same ratio applies throughout.

Step 4: Health expenditure savings

We can then scale this up to healthcare savings in general. In the UK, healthcare expenditure for 2013 came to a total of £124 billion (UK Public Spending, 2013). It follows from this that in a situation where companion animals did not exist in the UK, healthcare expenditure would have been:

$$£(82.5/80.9) \times 124 \text{ billion} = £126.45 \text{ billion}$$

Therefore, savings due to the existence of companion animals were:

$$£126.45 \text{ billion} - £124 \text{ billion} = £2.45 \text{ billion}$$

Through inserting UK health expenditure, population estimates and companion animal population estimates into an even more conservative framework than that presented in Headey (1998), it is suggested that for 2013, savings towards healthcare expenditure in the UK could have been in the region of £2.45 billion due to the existence of companion animals.

Clearly this is an approximate but conservative estimate, since it excludes benefits to other family members within the companion animal-owning household. On top of this, there is certainly further value for government and the UK economy arising from companion animal ownership associated with the reduced days off work in this population, but again these data are not currently available. Nonetheless this exercise serves to highlight the importance of further research on this matter, not only to provide a more accurate estimate of the economic impact of companion animal ownership on healthcare expenditure but also to assess the potential ways that companion animals may be used to improve human health and well-being to generate even greater societal and economic impact.

5B FURTHER VALUE – ANIMAL-ASSISTED INTERVENTIONS AND THE WIDER SUPPORT OF INDIVIDUALS WITH INCREASED NEED IN SOCIETY

Animal-assisted Interventions

Animal-assisted interventions (AAI) is a general term used to describe the variety of ways that companion animals can work with practitioners to enable the rehabilitation or social care of people and communities across a range of backgrounds.

It is not surprising that visiting or resident companion animals have been shown to have a positive impact on non-companion-animal owners. Several studies place a large emphasis on the effect of visiting dogs on the elderly population who reside in care homes and facilities (e.g. Salmon *et al.*, 1982; Crowley-Robinson *et al.*, 1996; Sellers, 2006).

Of the numerous studies, most employ the same technique of allowing one group (or more) of residents contact with a visiting dog and another no access (control group). Such procedures unsurprisingly lead to reports that those in contact with the visiting dog benefit from: (i) improvement in mental functioning (Kawamura *et al.*, 2007); (ii) reduced levels of loneliness (Banks & Banks, 2002, 2005; Banks *et al.*, 2008); and (iii) lower levels of depression (Le Roux & Kemp, 2009).

The introduction of a dog has been suggested to increase human inter-actions and contacts with other residents and staff. This is supported by studies comparing real and robotic dogs (Banks *et al.*, 2008; Kramer *et al.*, 2009). Interestingly, Banks *et al.* (2008) suggest that residents interacting with both a robotic dog and real dog not only report a reduction in lone-liness but also formed an attachment with both 'dogs', but the latter was not the cause of the reported lower levels of loneliness. Although the po-tential importance of dogs in providing social support is well recognized (e.g. Friedmann & Thomas, 1995; Antonacopoulos & Pychyl, 2008; Beetz *et al.*, 2012), it is worth noting that in relation to reducing loneliness, it has been found that interventions that address maladaptive cognitions are most effective (Masi *et al.*, 2010), and it is possible that dogs could serve this function too.

In addition to studies concentrating on the elderly in residential set-tings, there is a body of evidence suggesting that therapy dogs can help those who are hospitalized, including children, who may be stressed in hospital (e.g. Moody *et al.*, 2002; Bouchard *et al.*, 2004). As with those in care facilities, the dog could be seen as a cognitive distraction for indi-viduals, giving them something to functionally concentrate on and/or look forward to.

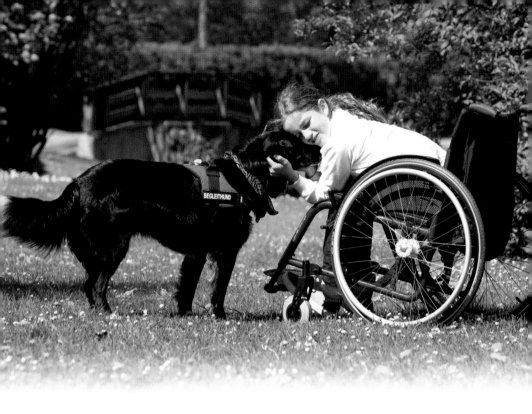

Assistance Dogs

The tangible benefits of a specific assistance animal are well known (e.g. dogs trained to provide assistance to client groups with a specific disability), but the scale, need and direct costs of the industry are perhaps less widely appreciated. Over recent years there has been a rise in the number and application of assistance dogs, and the organizations representing those with disabilities have grown tremendously.

In the UK (unlike some European countries), assistance dogs themselves are neither supplied nor supported by the government, but instead are often obtained by individuals through various charities whose purpose is to improve the lives of individuals with disabilities. Assistance Dogs (UK) (AD (UK)) is an umbrella organization within the UK representing seven assistance-dog organizations, with the purpose of encouraging 'the exchange of ideas and best practice among its members, rais[ing] awareness among the general public and promoting behavioural and legislative changes to ensure the freedom, independence and rights of its clients' (www.assistancedogs.org.uk). The seven registered organizations include the commonly known Guide Dogs and Hearing Dogs for Deaf People as well as Dogs for Good (formerly Dogs for the Disabled), Canine Partners, Support Dogs, Medical Detection Dogs and Dog Assistance in Disability (AID).

Within the UK, it is estimated that over 11 million people have a long-term illness, disability or impairment, equating to around 18% of the

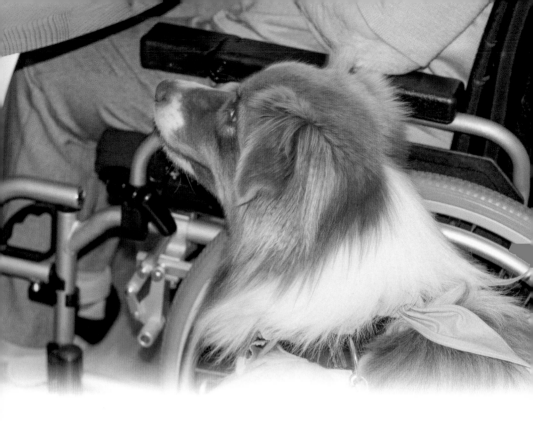

UK population (Family Resources Survey, 2008/09). Around 6% of children are disabled, while 16% of adults of working age and 45% of people over state pension age are disabled (Family Resources Survey, 2008/09). Over one-fifth of disabled people say that they do not frequently have choice and control over their daily lives and around one-third of disabled people experience difficulties related to their impairment in accessing public, commercial and leisure goods and services (Family Resources Survey, 2008/09). It is also acknowledged that those with disabilities remain significantly less likely to participate in cultural, leisure and sporting activities than non-disabled people (Taking Part Survey, 2009/10). Furthermore, 19.2% of working-age disabled people are reported as having no qualifications compared with 6.5% of non-disabled people, and only half of disabled people of working age are in work, compared with 80% of non-disabled people. There are currently 1.3 million disabled people in the UK who are available and want to work (Disability Living Facts, 2016). However, it is also noted that individuals with disabilities often experience discrimination in the workplace, with 19% of disabled people reportedly experiencing unfair treatment at work compared with 13% of non-disabled people (Fevre *et al.*, 2008).

The implications of disabilities are far more wide ranging than this to the individual. Many individuals with disabilities are dependent on others for care, usually in the form of paid and unpaid assistance from family and friends. In the UK, one in eight people – around 7 million – are carers, with an estimated 2 million people annually becoming care givers. Of these, around one in five carers is forced to give up work and 1.25 million people provide over 50 hours of care per week (www.carersuk.org). Over £5 billion is lost from the economy due to lost earnings from individuals giving up work to take on caring duties (www.carers.org). There are also a reported 21% of individuals in families with at least one disabled member living in relative income poverty (on a 'before housing costs' basis), compared with 16% of individuals in families with no disabled member (Department for Work and Pensions, 2011).

There are also sources of support from the government for people with disabilities, namely the Disability Living Allowance (DLA), or the Personal Independence Payment that is gradually replacing it. There are an estimated 3.27 million people claiming DLA (figures from November 2013; Department for Work and Pensions, 2014) and this appears to be a growing issue.

The Guide Dogs organization is involved in the training and supply of assistance dogs for the benefit of blind and partially sighted individuals. There are currently 370,000 people registered as blind or partially sighted in the UK, yet it is believed that almost 2 million people are living with sight loss in the UK (www.rnib.org.uk). Research by Guide Dogs suggests that 180,000 individuals who are blind or partially sighted rarely, if ever, leave their homes (Guide Dogs, 2010). It is estimated that indirect costs of sight loss, such as unpaid carer costs and reduced employment rates, total £5.3 billion (RNIB, 2013). The Guide Dogs organization currently supports 4700 guide-dog partnerships dogs, creating 800 new partnerships every year (Guide Dogs, 2013). It costs approximately £50,000 to support a guide dog from birth to retirement. The associated costs of breeding and puppy-walking dogs are approximately £3100 and £5100, respectively, while the cost of training guide dogs is £13,900 for basic and a further £10,100 for advanced training. There are also costs arising from creating the human–animal working partnership, calculated at £3300, and the financial contribution of supporting the partnership, calculated at £12,800. Overall, the Guide Dogs charity estimates that the cost of the core guide-dog service equates to £50 million/year (2012 figures; Guide Dogs, 2013).

Hearing Dogs for Deaf People trains dogs to alert individuals suffering from hearing loss to important sounds and danger signals in the home, workplace and public buildings. In 2011 there were estimated to be around 10 million people in the UK with some form of hearing loss, of which 800,000 people are severely or profoundly deaf (www.ActionHearingLoss.org.uk). Since 1982, Hearing Dogs for Deaf People has trained a total of 1600 dogs with 750 current working partnerships in the UK. Furthermore, the organization has jointly trained 14 dual-purpose dogs with other AD (UK)-accredited organizations, to meet the needs of those individuals with additional disabilities and requirements. The cost of a hearing dog is calculated at £45,000, which includes the associated costs of breeding, training, placement

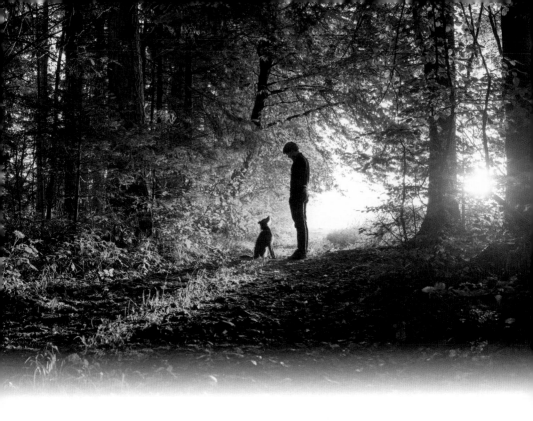

and life-long support of a human partnership (see Appendix Table 3; www. cabi.org/openresources/91728). Such figures would therefore suggest that the total value of providing current working partnerships stands at £33.75 million.

The mission of Support Dogs is 'to improve the quality of life for people with epilepsy, physical disabilities and children with autism by training dogs to act as safe and efficient assistants' (https://supportdogs. org.uk). The organization trains three categories of assistance dogs, which include disability assistance dogs, autism assistance dogs and seizure alert dogs, all of which are trained to fit the individual needs of the owners. To date, Support Dogs supports over 200 partnerships in the UK (Support Dogs, n.d.). It currently costs the organization over £30,000 to train a dog and support an assistance-dog partnership for life (see Appendix Table 4; www.cabi.org/openresources/91728). Such figures would therefore suggest that the total cost of providing current working partnerships stands at £6 million.

Canine Partners trains dogs to assist adults who have physical disabilities, with many of the clients being users of wheelchairs. The organization observes that around 1.2 million people currently use wheelchairs in the UK, of whom many would benefit from a canine partner. Their assistance dogs are trained to assist their owners' individual needs, which includes assisting with a range of practical tasks such as: (i) opening and shutting doors; (ii) retrieving objects; (iii) pressing buttons/switches; (iv) loading and unloading the washing machine; and (v) getting help in an emergency. In 2013 the organization supported 260 working partnerships, yet reportedly receives somewhere in the region of 400 enquires annually. The cost of creating a canine partnership stands at £20,000, which comprises selecting and training a dog, assessing the human applicant and also supporting the partnership for 10 years (see Appendix Table 4; www.cabi.org/openresources/91728). Such figures would therefore suggest that the direct investment made in providing these working partnerships stands at £5.2 million.

Communications with Medical Detection Dogs indicate that they have 60 dogs placed and in working partnerships across England, Wales and Scotland. They train Cancer Detection Dogs who can detect volatiles found in cancer cells, enabling scientists with the research and development of an early cancer screening system. As well as this, they train Medical Alert Dogs to empower individuals who manage complex medical conditions, for example identifying odour changes that are associated with certain medical events. The cost of training a Medical Detection Dog is around £11,200, including ongoing support (Medical Detection Dogs, 2016).

Dog AID is of relatively small size in comparison to the others, yet no less important. This organization differentiates itself from others as it allows a disabled owner to train their own dog to assist in their additional needs. Little information and few figures are available for this non-profit organization, except that all the trainers are volunteers and the demand for service is demonstrated by potential clients being put on to a 1–2 year waiting list.

Dogs for Good (formerly Dogs for the Disabled) trains assistance dogs for children and adults with physical disabilities as well as assistance dogs for families with a child with autism and more broadly supports canine-assisted interventions. It is difficult to obtain accurate information on the number of people with autism in the UK, yet it is estimated that there are probably more than half a million, so consequently more than 2 million people are affected when family members are taken into consideration (www.autism.org.uk). In 2012, Dogs for the Disabled (as they were) created 47 new assistance-dog partnerships, with 28 adults and 10 children with physical disabilities benefitting, as well as nine children affected by autism. The overall number of assistance dogs supported by Dogs for Good currently totals 275: 180 assistance-dog partnerships for adults with physical disabilities, 56 assistance-dog teams for children with disabilities and a further 39 assistance dogs for children affected by autism. The cost of an assistance-dog partnership is approximately £20,000, which is based on the cost of training an 8-week-old puppy to become a fully qualified assistance dog (£12,000), as well as creating and supporting the partnership throughout its lifetime (Dogs for Good, n.d.). It is therefore calculated that the total value of providing current working partnerships stands at around £5.5 million, with the charity having annual running costs of £3 million.

There is a growing body of research on the benefits of assistance and family dogs to families and children affected by autism. Children with autism can display unpredictable and volatile behaviour, which can place them in danger, as well as causing great stress for a family. A small-scale study (Burrows et al., 2008) found that incorporating an assistance dog into a family with a child with autism produced positive outcomes on the behaviour of the children with autism, enhancing safety, relieving stress of family members and enhancing activities and outings for the family, which would otherwise not have occurred in the absence of the assistance dog. In recognition that many of the benefits of an assistance dog to an autistic child may extend from the companionship provided, and to increase accessibility of its services, Dogs for Good has been working with dogs in the home through the PAWS (Parents Autism Workshops & Support) service. Since launching this service in 2010, Dogs for Good has been able to support a further 500 families affected by autism, by hosting a series of workshops alongside aftercare to assist families in managing and training their own dog for their child affected by autism. Results from a longitudinal study of these families in association with the University of Lincoln suggest that the benefits of dog ownership are not only reaped by the child, but that there are also significant changes in the mental health of their primary carers and that they are sustained over a 3-year period (Wright et al., 2015a,b; Hall et al., 2016). At a time when the health of this population (unpaid carers) is of growing political concern, this deserves closer attention.

Consideration should be paid to the fact that children with autism grow up to be adults with autism, and therefore are still potentially dependent on others. Within the UK there are no charities that specifically support canine partnerships for adults with autism. Furthermore, the topic of autism assistance dogs seems relatively unexplored, even by the National Autistic Society. Despite this, the topic seems to be the focus of numerous online support chat rooms for adults with autism. During the course of developing this report, one online discussion, found at www.ambitiousaboutautism.org.uk, was of particular interest. The topic of the discussion was assistance dogs for adults with autism in the workplace. The conversation covered a variety of subjects including from where to source assistance dogs by individual financing and the issue of these dogs not having the access rights that other assistance dogs have. Potential benefits of autism dogs for adults that were highlighted consisted of: (i) enhanced social support; (ii) a way of calming down; (iii) helping to break out of over-focusing; and (iv) helping individuals learn about relationships. While not necessarily stating that assistance dogs have enabled greater employment, it is assumed that dogs could be beneficial in the workplace. Indeed, only 15% of adults with autism are in full-time employment, yet most are in fact willing and able to work (www.autism.org.uk).

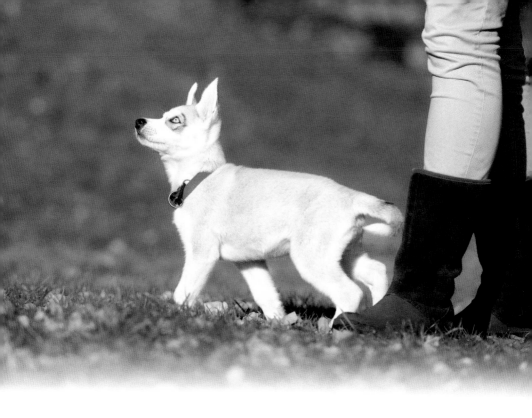

Classroom Dogs

The value of animals in the classroom is of increasing interest to schools across the UK, yet much of this work is unmoderated and not validated, making it difficult to obtain figures on the number of classroom animals, their purpose and their effects. Nonetheless, reports indicate that reading to dog programmes, such as the Kennel Club's Bark and Read project, improve children's motivation and interest in reading (Intermountain Therapy Animals, 2011; Friesen & Delisle, 2012; Shaw, 2013; The Kennel Club, 2016). It is estimated that poor literacy skills cost the UK over £2 billion a year (National Literacy Trust, 2009). However, over the past decade there has been a worrying decline in children's enjoyment, and therefore frequency, of reading (Sainsbury & Schagen, 2004). Given that frequency of reading is directly related to reading attainment (Clark & Douglas, 2011), it is recognized by government that it is essential that we implement strategies to improve children's reading motivation and enjoyment to encourage more regular reading (Department for Education, 2012), and dogs may prove an economically valid tool to achieving this.

Additionally, there is much anecdotal evidence to support the use of dogs in the classroom to reduce truancy (Pets in the Classroom, 2015). School truancy is strongly related to youth crime and youth unemployment (Prince's Trust, 2007). In 2004 youth crimes cost the UK over £1 billion. The daily cost of youth unemployment to the UK due to productivity loss is £10 million, and with £20 million a week added on due to benefit payments the

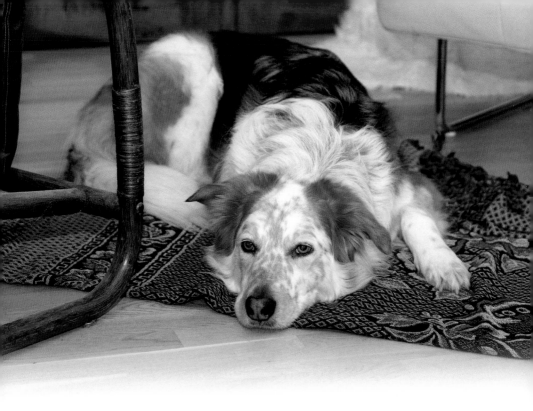

monthly cost is £360 million (Prince's Trust, 2007). Yet again it is clear that the use of dogs in the classroom has the potential to make wide-reaching positive impacts on the UK economy, but until these qualitative trends can be quantified and explored in detail, recommendations cannot be implemented into educational policies.

Recognizing the Value of such Programmes

Studies and literature detailing mechanisms by which assistance dogs help and benefit those with disabilities appear to be relatively limited. The probable reason for this is likely to be the subjective nature and complexity of benefits, as well as limited funding opportunities. Issues also occur in generalizing benefits, which is undoubtedly why individual case studies are often used to demonstrate the potential benefits (e.g. Duncan & Allen, 2001). The studies that do exist tend to be from countries other than the UK, and also have relatively small numbers of participants. However, this is not surprising considering the actual number of working partnerships that currently exist. Outcomes of assistance-animal partnerships are normally concluded from self-report questionnaires completed by the participants during studies.

Potential benefits of economic significance include indirect effects on others, for example by providing enhanced independent living; through helping with practical tasks, the individual is less dependent on family, friends and employed helpers. It should also be noted that the work done by an assistance dog helps to limit potential risks and injuries for their human partner. Furthermore, because dogs have public access rights it enables owners to have greater practical opportunities to take part in events and have greater engagement with the community and service industries.

While the primary purpose of an assistance dog is often to enhance the physical capabilities of their owners, it should be noted that the nature of the dog's presence can also give an individual companionship through sharing everyday life events with someone, as well as possibly facilitating greater social interaction. Studies have seemed to support this notion, with early studies observing that adults with assistance dogs report a significantly higher number of social greetings, acknowledgement and approaches in public places than those without an assistance dog (Hart *et al.*, 1987; Eddy *et al.*, 1988), and the same is also suggested for children with assistance dogs (Mader *et al.*, 1989). Further studies indicate that individuals with assistance dogs report substantial improvement in self-esteem, internal locus of control, psychological well-being and improved social aspects through greater community integration (Allen & Blascovich, 1996).

Developing a Case for Economic Benefit

Within the available literature, it is clear that assistance partnerships bring wider economic benefits. One of the more important economic impacts associated with obtaining an assistance dog might be a reduction in human assistance hours. One such study by Allen and Blascovich (1996), of individuals with ambulatory disabilities, reported that the acquisition of an assistance dog resulted in a reduction of approximately 60 (68%) bi-weekly paid assistance hours and a further reduction of approximately 25 (64%) bi-weekly unpaid assistance hours, thus 'diminishing a substantial time and economic burden for family and friends who were care givers' (p. 1004). Furthermore, increases in school attendances and part-time work were also associated with acquiring an assistance dog. Increases in employment are also acknowledged by Duncan and Allen (2001), who report the impact of assistance dogs on employment through case studies. Such case studies indicate a possible means for ensuring that a person's disability does not adversely affect their work. It has also been noted that the presence of an assistance dog has a positive impact on the feelings of the employer that an individual can capably perform in their job role. Furthermore, it is also suggested that assistance dogs aid and enable an individual to use public transport, therefore actually enabling an individual to get to work.

Many of the studies and examples already listed suggest that individuals with assistance dogs may be far less dependent on others for transport and have greater independent mobility. However, the effect on use of private or

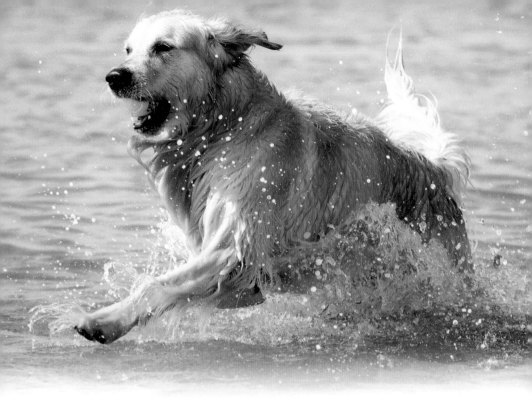

public transport has been relatively unexplored. An increase in the use of public transport by those with disabilities, more so within the UK, could also create economic savings for the individual and local authorities and requires further exploration and investigation.

The perceived outcome associated with the acquisition of an assistance dog needs further study, particularly in the way assistance dogs actually contribute to reduction in paid human assistance hours. Indeed, without knowing exactly how the presence of an assistance dog facilitates these outcomes, it could be assumed that the benefits are just psychological (see Coppinger, 1998). As observed by Duncan and Allen (2001), 'Although there are many anecdotal reports documenting the instrumental and emotional support provided by service [assistance] animals, little research has systematically addressed the degree to which such animals can actually change the lives of people with disabilities', and this is still the same situation 15 years on.

Conclusion: Illustrating the Perceived Economic Impact of Companion Animals

6

There is overwhelming evidence to suggest that companion animals have a significant economic impact on the UK economy; however, the scale of this remains uncertain in terms of both the range of mechanisms involved and the monetary value of these. This report has sought to highlight both of these matters with a view to increasing awareness of these issues and the need for further research in this area. We do not believe it is acceptable to simply dismiss the lack of high-quality evidence as demonstrating a lack of effect or importance of this topic. As mentioned earlier, from an economic perspective it is important to consider the cost of failing to act versus acting on what is suggested by the literature. In our opinion, at a time of fiscal constraints, there is a greater need to explore the potential saving that could be made through low-cost interventions such as the greater exploitation of the value of companion animals in society, and the cost of any legislation that potentially limits this should be appreciated.

It is also important to appreciate that when examining complex and dynamic issues like the impact of companion animals on individual health and well-being, there may be multiple mechanisms involved that operate at different times on different individuals according to their circumstances. This poses scientific challenges, but does not mean research in this area need be unscientific. Perhaps the main barrier to good-quality scientific research is the availability of funding. From an economic perspective, the impacts can be divided into direct and indirect, and examples of both have been given in this report.

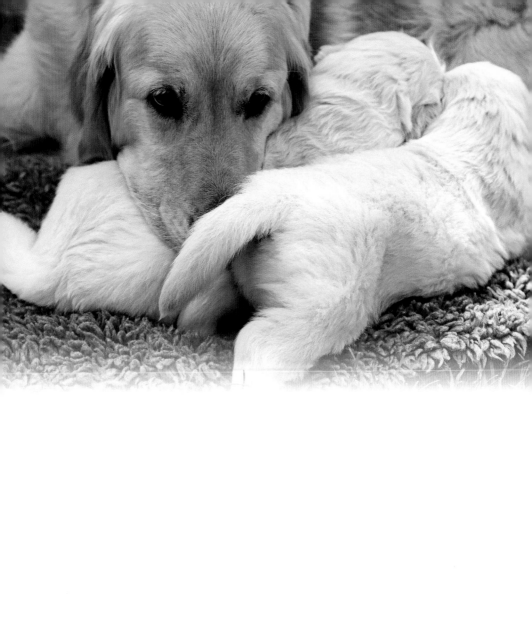

Acknowledgement

We are very grateful to the WALTHAM Centre for Pet Nutrition for contributing to the scope and content of this report and for supplying the photographs. We also thank Mars Petcare UK for their generous sponsorship towards the cost of producing the report.

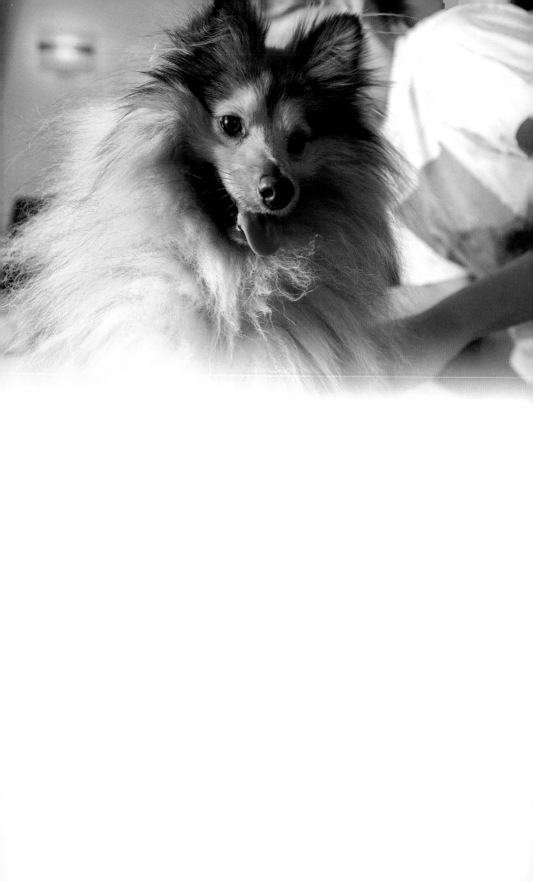

Afterword

Mars Petcare UK is delighted to have had the opportunity to be involved in the development of *Companion Animal Economics: The Economic Impact of Companion Animals in the UK*. This timely report provides a much-needed update on the previous Council for Science and Society (CSS) report *Companion Animals in Society*, which dates back to 1988. In the intervening period the UK has become an increasingly ageing society, with people too often isolated by the increasing digitalization of communications. In this context, the value of pets in combating isolation and loneliness has never been more important.

At Mars Petcare UK our driving ambition is: A BETTER WORLD FOR PETS™. Individually we all love and cherish our pets, but we rarely stop to consider why this is, how we can make the most of our relationships with them and how others too might benefit.

It is vital that we acknowledge just how much comfort and companionship pets can provide when we are lonely, how much joy they can bring when we are depressed and how much assistance they can offer to those who need a helping hand. Ultimately, pets can be a lifeline to those in need. It is high time that we properly assess and measure this support, to address the costs of pet ownership while preserving the significant potential savings on healthcare costs across the UK's public services.

Shining a well-deserved spotlight on this economic value is what this report has tried to do. And this is only the beginning. It is my hope that the findings of this report will prompt further research in this area and lead to a better understanding of the value of our pets to individuals and to all of society. I sincerely hope that policy makers take notice of these lessons and that, in the future, the full benefits of pet ownership are recognized, appreciated and fully encouraged.

Damian Guha
Managing Director
Mars Petcare UK

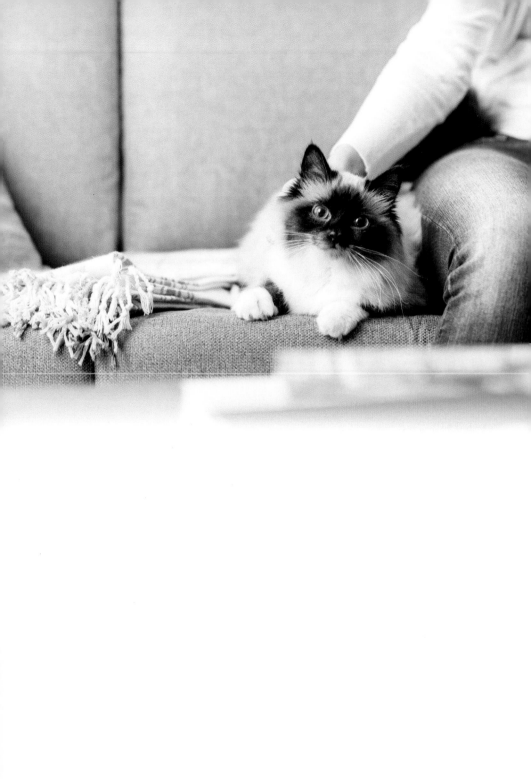

References

Adkins, S.L. & Rajecki, D.W. (1999). Pets' roles in parents' bereavement. *Anthrozoös: A Multidisciplinary Journal of the Interactions of People & Animals*, 12(1), 33–42.

Akiyama, H., Holtzman, J.M. & Britz, W.E. (1987). Pet ownership and health status during bereavement. *OMEGA – Journal of Death and Dying*, 17(2), 187–193.

Allen, K.M. (2001). Dog ownership and control of borderline hypertension: a controlled randomized trial. Presented at the 22nd Annual Scientific Sessions of the Society of Behavioural Medicine, Seattle, Washington, March 2001.

Allen, K.M. (2003). Are pets a healthy pleasure? The influence of pets on blood pressure. *Current Directions in Psychological Science*, 12(6), 236–239.

Allen, K.M. & Blascovich, J. (1996). The value of service dogs for people with severe ambulatory disabilities: a randomized, controlled trial. *Journal of the American Medical Association*, 275(13), 1001–1006.

Allen, K.M., Blascovich, J., Tomaka, J. & Kelsey, R.M. (1991). Presence of human friends and pet dogs as moderators of autonomic responses to stress in women. *Journal of Personality and Social Psychology*, 61(4), 582–589.

American Veterinary Medical Association (AVMA) (2006). Human–Animal Bond. Available at: https://www.avma.org/kb/resources/reference/human-animal-bond/pages/human-animal-bond-avma.aspx (accessed 3 March 2016).

Anderson, W.P., Reid, C.M. & Jennings, G.L. (1992). Pet ownership and risk factors for cardiovascular disease. *Medical Journal of Australia*, 157(5), 298–301.

Antonacopoulos, N.M.D. & Pychyl, T.A. (2008). An examination of the relations between social support, anthropomorphism and stress among dog owners. *Anthrozoös*, 21(2), 139–152.

Antonacopoulos, N.M.D. & Pychyl, T.A. (2010). An examination of the potential role of pet ownership, human social support and pet attachment in the psychological health of individuals living alone. *Anthrozoös*, 23(1), 37–54.

Association of British Insurers (2015). Insurers now paying out £1.65m a day to treat the nation's pets. Available at: https://www.abi.org.uk/News/News releases/2015/05/Insurers-now-paying-out-1-65m-a-day-to-treat-the-nations-pets (accessed 31 May 2016).

Banks, M.R. & Banks, W.A. (2002). The effects of animal-assisted therapy on loneliness in an elderly population in long-term care facilities. *Journal of Gerontology: Medical Sciences*, 57, 428–432.

Banks, M.R. & Banks, W.A. (2005). The effects of group and individual animal-assisted therapy on loneliness in residents of long-term care facilities. *Anthrozoös*, 18(4), 396–408.

Banks, M.R., Willoughby, L.M. & Banks, W.A. (2008). Animal-assisted therapy and loneliness in nursing homes: use of robotic versus living dogs. *Journal of the American Medical Directors Association*, 9(3), 173–177.

Barker, S.B. & Wolen, A.R. (2008). The benefits of human–companion animal interaction: a review. *Journal of Veterinary Medical Education*, 35(4), 487–495.

Barker, S.B., Knisley, J.S., McCain, N.L., Schubert, C.M. & Pandurangi, A.K. (2010). Exploratory study of stress buffering response patterns from interaction with a therapy dog. *Anthrozoös*, 23, 79–91.

Battersea (2010). Celebrating our past, safeguarding our future. 150th Anniversary Year Annual Review 2010. Available at: http://www.bdch.org.uk/files/AR2010.pdf (accessed 31 May 2016).

Battersea (2014). Battersea Dogs & Cats Home Annual Review 2014. Available at: http://www.bdch.org.uk/files/AR2014.pdf (accessed 31 May 2016).

Bauman, A.E., Russell, S.J., Furber, S.E. & Dobson, A.J. (2001). The epidemiology of dog walking: an unmet need for human and canine health. *Medical Journal of Australia*, 175(11/12), 632–634.

Baun, M.M., Bergstrom, N., Langston, N.F. & Thoma, L. (1984). Physiological effects of human/companion animal bonding. *Nursing Research*, 33(3), 126–129.

Beetz, A., Julius, H., Turner, D. & Kotrschal, K. (2012). Effects of social support by a dog on stress modulation in male children with insecure attachment. *Frontiers in Psychology*, 3, 352. Available at: http://doi.org/10.3389/fpsyg.2012.00352 (accessed 2 September 2016).

Bennett, P.C., Trigg, J.L., Godber, T. & Brown, C. (2015). An experience sampling approach to investigating associations between pet presence and indicators of psychological wellbeing and mood in older Australians. *Anthrozoös*, 28(3), 403–420.

Bennett, T. & Wright, R. (1984). What the burglar saw. *New Society*, 67(1106), 162–163.

Berget, B. & Grepperud, S. (2011). Animal-assisted interventions for psychiatric patients: beliefs in treatment effects among practitioners. *European Journal of Integrative Medicine*, 3(2), e91–e96.

Bergroth, E., Remes, S., Pekkanen, J., Kauppila, T., Büchele, G. & Keski-Nisula, L. (2012). Respiratory tract illnesses during the first year of life: effect of dog and cat contacts. *Pediatrics for Parents*, 130(2), 211–220.

Black, K. (2012). The relationship between companion animals and loneliness among rural adolescents. *Journal of Pediatric Nursing*, 27(2), 103–112.

Bouchard, F., Landry, M., Belles-Isles, M. & Gagnon, J. (2004). A magical dream: a pilot project in animal-assisted therapy in pediatric oncology. *Canadian Oncology Nursing Journal*, 14, 14–17.

Burrows, K.E., Adams, C.L. & Spiers, J. (2008). Sentinels of safety: service dogs ensure safety and enhance freedom and well-being for families with autistic children. *Qualitative Health Research*, 18(12), 1642–1649.

Bustad, L.K. (1980). *Animals, Aging and the Aged*. University of Minnesota Press, Minneapolis, Minnesota.

Bustad, L.K. & Hines, L.M. (1983). Placement of animals with the elderly: benefits and strategies. In A.H. Katcher & A.M. Beck (Eds), *New Perspectives on our Lives with Companion Animals*. University of Pennsylvania Press, Philadelphia, Pennsylvania, pp. 291–302.

Cain, A.O. (1985). Pets as family members. *Marriage & Family Review*, 8(3–4), 5–10.

Carlsen, K.C.L., Roll, S., Carlsen, K.H., Mowinckel, P., Wijga, A.H., Brunekreef, B., Torrent, M., Roberts, G., Arshad, S.H., Kull, I. & Krämer, U. (2012). Does pet ownership in infancy lead to asthma or allergy at school age? Pooled analysis of individual participant data from 11 European birth cohorts. *PLoS ONE*, 7(8), e43214.

Carmack, B.J. (1991). The role of companion animals for persons with AIDS/HIV. *Holistic Nursing Practice*, 5(2), 24–31.

Castelli, P., Hart, L.A. & Zasloff, R.L. (2001). Companion cats and the social support systems of men with AIDS. *Psychological Reports*, 89(1), 177–187.

Cats Protection (2014). Cats Protection 2014 Annual Review. Available at: http://www.cats.org.uk/uploads/documents/Annual_Review_2014_web_version.pdf (accessed 31 May 2016).

Christian, H.E., Westgarth, C., Bauman, A., Richards, E.A., Rhodes, R., Evenson, K.R., Mayer, J.A. & Thorpe, R.J. (2013). Dog ownership and physical activity: a review of the evidence. *Journal of Physical Activity and Health*, 10(5), 750–759.

Clark, C. & Douglas, J. (2011). *Young People's Reading and Writing: an In-depth Study Focusing on Enjoyment, Behaviour, Attitudes and Attainment*. National Literacy Trust, London.

Clower, T.L. & Neaves, T.T. (2015). The Health Care Cost Savings of Pet Ownership. HABRI report. Available at: http://habri.org/docs/HABRI_Report_-_Healthcare_Cost_Savings_from_Pet_Ownership_.pdf (accessed 15 September 2016).

Coleman, K.J., Rosenberg, D.E., Conway, T.L., Sallis, J.F., Saelens, B.E., Frank, L.D. & Cain, K. (2008). Physical activity, weight status, and neighbourhood characteristics of dog walkers. *Preventive Medicine*, 47(3), 309–312.

Coppinger, R. (1998). Breeding, training and the use of service/assistance dogs: a positive critique. Presented as a plenary address at the 8th International Conference on Human–Animal Interactions, 'The Changing Roles of Animals in Society', Prague, Czech Republic, September 1998.

Council for Science and Society (CSS) (1988). *Companion Animals in Society: Report of a Working Party*. Oxford University Press, New York.

Crossman, M.K. & Kazdin, A.E. (2016). Additional evidence is needed to recommend acquiring a dog to families of children with autism spectrum disorder: a response to Wright and colleagues. *Journal of Autism and Developmental Disorders*, 46(1), 332–335.

Crowley-Robinson, P., Fenwick, D. & Blackshaw, J. (1996). A long-term study of elderly people in nursing homes with visiting and resident dogs. *Applied Animal Science*, 47, 137–148.

Cutt, H. (2007). The effect of walking the dog on adult physical activity levels: implications for local and state government. In *Proceedings of People, Pets and Planning Symposium: Living in a Healthy Community*. Deakin University, Melbourne, Australia, November 2007, pp. 19–21.

Cutt, H., Giles-Corti, B., Knuiman, M., Timperio, A. & Bull, F.C. (2008). Understanding dog owners' increased levels of physical activity: results from RESIDE. *American Journal of Public Health*, 98(1), 66–69.

Davis, K.L. & Belnap, C.S. (2013). Pets at birth do not increase allergic disease in at-risk children. *Pediatrics*, 132(Supplement 1), S5–S5.

Department for Education (2012). Research evidence on reading for pleasure. Available at: https://www.gov.uk/government/uploads/system/uploads/attachment_data/file/284286/reading_for_pleasure.pdf (accessed 3 March 2016).

Department for Work and Pensions (2011). Households Below Average Income: An analysis of the income distribution 1994/95 – 2009/10, May 2011. Available at: https://www.gov.uk/government/uploads/system/uploads/attachment_data/file/211950/full_hbai11.pdf (accessed 31 May 2016).

Department for Work and Pensions (2014). DWP Quarterly Statistical Summary. Available at: https://www.gov.uk/government/uploads/system/uploads/attachment_data/file/382255/stats_summary_may14_final_v1.pdf (accessed 31 May 2016).

Department of Health (2013). Reference costs 2012-13. Available at: https://www.gov.uk/government/uploads/system/uploads/attachment_data/file/261154/nhs_reference_costs_2012-13_acc.pdf (accessed 31 May 2016).

Dietz, T.J., Davis, D. & Pennings, J. (2012). Evaluating animal-assisted therapy in group treatment for child sexual abuse. *Journal of Child Sexual Abuse*, 21(6), 665–683.

Disability Living Facts (2016). Key facts. Available at: http://www.dlf.org.uk/content/key-facts (accessed 31 May 2016).

Dogs for Good (n.d.). About the Charity. Available at: https://www.dogsforgood.org/media-centre/press-office/about-the-charity-2/ (accessed 31 May 2016).

Duncan, S.L. & Allen, K. (2001). Service animals and their roles in enhancing independence, quality of life, and employment for people with disabilities. In A.H. Fine (Ed.), *Handbook on Animal-assisted Therapy: Theoretical Foundations and Guidelines for Practice*. Academic Press, San Diego, California, pp. 303–324.

Eddy, J., Hart, L.A. & Boltz, R.P. (1988). The effects of service dogs on social acknowledgement of people in wheelchairs. *The Journal of Psychology*, 122, 39–45.

Esteves, S.W. & Stokes, T. (2008). Social effects of a dog's presence on children with disabilities. *Anthrozoös*, 21, 5–15.

Family Resources Survey (2008/09). Available at: http://webarchive.nationalarchives.gov.uk/20120930153352/http://statistics.dwp.gov.uk/asd/frs/2008_09/index.php?page=intro (accessed 15 September 2016).

Fevre, R., Nichols, T., Prior, G. & Rutherford, I. (2008). Fair Treatment at Work Survey. Available at: https://www.gov.uk/government/uploads/system/uploads/attachment_data/file/192191/09-P85-fair-treatment-at-work-report-2008-survey-errs-103.pdf (accessed 31 May 2016).

Fine, A.H. (Ed.) (2010). *Handbook on Animal-assisted Therapy: Theoretical Foundations and Guidelines for Practice*. Academic Press, San Diego, California.

Friedmann, E. & Lockwood, R. (1993). Perception of animals and cardiovascular responses during verbalization with an animal present. *Anthrozoös*, 6, 115–134.

Friedmann, E. & Thomas, S.A. (1995). Pet ownership, social support, and one-year survival after acute myocardial infarction in the Cardiac Arrhythmia Suppression Trial (CAST). *The American Journal of Cardiology*, 76(17), 1213–1217.

Friedmann, E., Katcher, A.H., Lynch, J.J. & Thomas, S.A. (1980). Animal companions and one-year survival of patients after discharge from a coronary care unit. *Public Health Reports*, 95(4), 307–312.

Friedmann, E., Thomas, S.A., Cook, L.K., Chia-Chun, T. & Picot, S.J. (2007). A friendly dog as potential moderator of cardiovascular response to speech in older hypertensives. *Anthrozoös*, 20(1), 51–63.

Friesen, L. & Delisle, E. (2012). Animal-assisted literacy: a supportive environment for constrained and unconstrained learning. *Childhood Education*, 88, 102–107.

Garrity, T.F., Stallones, L., Marx, M.B. & Johnson, T.P. (1989). Pet ownership and attachment as supportive factors in the health of the elderly. *Anthrozoös*, 3(1), 35–44.

Gee, N.R., Sherlock, T.R., Bennett, E.A. & Harris, S.L. (2009). Preschoolers' adherence to instructions as a function of presence of a dog and motor skills task. *Anthrozoös*, 22, 267–276.

Gov.uk (2016). Controlling your dog in public: 4. Dog fouling. Available at: https://www.gov.uk/control-dog-public/dog-fouling (accessed 31 May 2016).

Guardabassi, L., Schwarz, S. & Lloyd, D.H. (2004). Pet animals as reservoirs of antimicrobial-resistant bacteria: review. *Journal of Antimicrobial Chemotherapy*, 54(2), 321–332.

Guéguen, N. & Ciccotti, S. (2008). Domestic dogs as facilitators in social interaction: an evaluation of helping and courtship behaviors. *Anthrozoös*, 21(4), 339–349.

Guide Dogs (2010). The Guide Dogs for the Blind Association Report and Financial Statements 2010. Available at: https://www.guidedogs.org.uk/media/1396823/Annual_Report_and_Accounts.pdf (accessed 31 May 2016).

Guide Dogs (2013). Cost of a guide dog. Available at: http://www.guidedogs.org.uk/media/3701632/Cost-of-a-guide-dog-2013.pdf (accessed 31 May 2016).

Hall, S., Wright, H., Hames, A., PAWS Team & Mills, D.S. (2016). The long-term benefits of dog ownership in families with children with autism. *Journal of Veterinary Behavior and Clinical Applications and Research*, 13, 46–54.

Ham, S.A. & Epping, J. (2006). Dog walking and physical activity in the United States. *Preventing Chronic Disease*, 3(2). Available at: http://www.cdc.gov/pcd/issues/2006/apr/05_0106.htm (accessed 7 February 2016).

Hart, L.A., Hart, B.L. & Bergin, B. (1987). Socializing effects of service dogs for people with disabilities. *Anthrozoös*, 1, 41–44.

Headey, B. (1995). Health benefits of pets: results from the Australian People and Pets Survey. Presented at the Urban Animal Management Conference, Australia, 1995.

Headey, B. (1998). Health benefits and health cost savings due to pets. *Social Indicators Research*, 47, 233–243.

Headey, B. & Anderson, W. (1995). *Health Cost Savings. The Impact of Pets on the Australian Health Budget*. Baker Medical Research Institute, The Centre for Public Policy, The University of Melbourne. November 1995. Petcare Information and Advisory Service, Wodonga, Victoria, Australia.

Headey, B. & Grabka, M.M. (2007). Pets and human health in Germany and Australia: national longitudinal results. *Social Indicators Research*, 80(2), 297–311.

Headey, B., Na, F. & Zheng, R. (2008). Pet dogs benefit owners' health: a 'natural experiment' in China. *Social Indicators Research*, 87(3), 481–493.

Health & Social Care Information Centre (HSCIC) (2014). Dog bites: hospital admissions in most deprived areas three times as high as least deprived. Available at: http://www.hscic.gov.uk/article/4722/Dog-bites-hospital-admissions-in-most-deprived-areas-three-times-as-high-as-least-deprived (accessed 31 May 2016).

Herzog, H. (2011). The impact of pets on human health and psychological well-being: fact, fiction, or hypothesis? *Current Directions in Psychological Science*, 20(4), 236–239.

Herzog, H. (2016). Three reasons why pets don't lower health care costs. Available at: https://www.psychologytoday.com/blog/animals-and-us/201601/three-reasons-why-pets-dont-lower-health-care-costs (accessed 31 May 2016).

Hesselmar, B., Aberg, N., Aberg, B., Eriksson, B. & Bjorksten, B. (1999). Does early exposure to cat or dog protect against later allergy development? *Clinical and Experimental Allergy*, 29, 611–617.

Heyworth, J.S., Cutt, H. & Glonek, G. (2006). Does dog or cat ownership lead to increased gastroenteritis in young children in South Australia? *Epidemiology and Infection*, 134(5), 926–934.

Hippisley-Cox, J. & Vinogradova, Y. (2009). Trends in Consultation Rates in General Practice 1995 to 2008: Analysis of the QResearch® database. Available at: http://www.hscic.gov.uk/catalogue/PUB01077/tren-cons-rate-gene-prac-95-09-95-08-rep.pdf (accessed 31 May 2016).

IBIS World (2011). Veterinary Services Market Research Report. Available at: http://www.ibisworld.co.uk/market-research/veterinary-services.html (accessed 31 May 2016).

Intermountain Therapy Animals (2011). R.E.A.D. Available at: http://www.therapyanimals.org/R.E.A.D.html (accessed 10 December 2013).

Karimi, M., Mirzaei, M., Baghiani Moghadam, B., Fotouhi, E. & Zare Mehrjardi, A. (2011). Pet exposure and the symptoms of asthma, allergic rhinitis and eczema in 6–7 years old children. *Iranian Journal of Asthma, Allergies and Immunology*, 10(2), 123–127.

Katcher, A.H. (1981). Interaction between people and their pets: form and function. In B. Fogle (Ed.), *Interrelations Between People and Pets*. Charles C. Thomas, Springfield, Illinois, pp. 42–67.

Katcher, A.H., Friedmann, E., Beck, A.M. & Lynch, J.J. (1983). Talking, looking and blood pressure: physiological consequences of interaction with the living environment. In A.H. Katcher & A.M. Bell (Eds), *New Perspectives on our Lives with Companion Animals*. University of Pennsylvania Press, Philadelphia, Pennsylvania, pp. 351–359.

Kawamura, N., Niiyama, M. & Niiyama, H. (2007). Long-term evaluation of animal-assisted therapy for institutionalized elderly people. *Psychogeriatrics*, 7, 8–13.

Kikusui, T., Winslow, J.T. & Mori, Y. (2006). Social buffering: relief from stress and anxiety. *Philosophical Transactions of the Royal Society B (Biological Sciences)*, 361(1476), 2215–2228.

Knight, S. & Edwards, V. (2008). In the company of wolves: the physical, social and psychological benefits of dog ownership. *Journal of Aging and Health*, 20, 437–455.

Koivusilta, L.K. & Ojanlatva, A. (2006). To have or not to have a pet for better health? *PLoS ONE*, 1(1), e109.

Kramer, S.C., Friedmann, E. & Bernstein, P.L. (2009). Comparison of the effect of human interaction, animal-assisted therapy, and AIBO-assisted therapy on long-term care residents with dementia. *Anthrozoös*, 22(1), 43–57.

Lang, U.E., Jansen, J.B., Wertenauer, F., Gallinat, J. & Rapp, M.A. (2010). Reduced anxiety during dog assisted interviews in acute schizophrenic patients. *European Journal of Integrative Medicine*, 2(3), 123–127.

Lantra (2010). Environmental and land-based industries. The sector skills council for environmental and land-based industries. Available at: http://www2.warwick.ac.uk/fac/soc/ier/ngrf/lmifuturetrends/sectorscovered/agriculture/lantra_aacs_lmi_march__2010.pdf (accessed 7 February 2016).

Le Roux, M.C. & Kemp, R. (2009). Effect of a companion dog on depression, and anxiety levels of elderly residents in a long-term care facility. *Psychogeriatrics*, 9(1), 23–26.

Levine, G.N., Allen, K., Braun, L.T., Christian, H.E., Friedmann, E., Taubert, K.A., Thomas S.A., Wells, D.L. & Lange, R.A. (2013). Pet ownership and cardiovascular risk a scientific statement from the American Heart Association. *Circulation*, 127(23), 2353–2363.

Levinson, B.M. (1972). *Pets and Human Development*. Charles C. Thomas, Springfield, Illinois.

Lodge, C.J., Allen, K.J., Lowe, A.J., Hill, D.J., Hosking, C.S., Abramson, M.J. & Dharmage, S.C. (2011). Perinatal cat and dog exposure and the risk of asthma and allergy in the urban environment: a systematic review of longitudinal studies. *Clinical and Developmental Immunology*, 176484. Available at: http://dx.doi.org/10.1155/2012/176484 (accessed 2 September 2016).

Mader, M., Hart L. & Bergin, B. (1989). Social acknowledgements for children with disabilities: effects of service dogs. *Child Development*, 60, 1529–1534.

Masi, C.M., Chen, H.Y., Hawkley, L.C. & Cacioppo, J.T. (2010). A meta-analysis of interventions to reduce loneliness. *Personality and Social Psychology Review*, 15(3), doi: 10.1177/1088868310377394.

McConnell, A.R., Brown, C.M., Shoda, T.M., Stayton, L.E. & Martin, C.E. (2011). Friends with benefits: on the positive consequences of pet ownership. *Journal of Personality and Social Psychology*, 101(6), 1239–1259.

McCrone, P., Dhanasiri, S., Patel, A., Knapp, M. & Lawton-Smith, S. (2008). *Paying the Price. The Cost of Mental Health Care in England to 2026*. Kings Fund, London.

McNicholas, J. & Collis, G.M. (2000). Dogs as catalysts for social interactions: robustness of the effect. *British Journal of Psychology*, 91(1), 61–70.

McNicholas, J. & Collis, G.M. (2001). Children's representations of pets in their social networks. *Child: Care, Health and Development*, 27(3), 279–294.

McNicholas, J., Collis, G.M., Kent, C. & Rogers, M. (2001). The role of pets in the support networks of people recovering from breast cancer. Presented at the 9th International Conference on Human–Animal Interactions, 'People and Animals, A Global Perspective for the 21st Century', Brazil, September 2001.

McNicholas, J., Gilbey, A., Rennie, A., Ahmedzai, S., Dono, J.A. & Ormerod, E. (2005). Pet ownership and human health: a brief review of evidence and issues. *British Medical Journal*, 331(7527), 1252–1254.

Medical Detection Dogs (2016). About Medical Detection Dogs. Available at: http://www.medicaldetectiondogs.org.uk/general_faqs.html (accessed 31 May 2016).

Mills, D.S. & De Keuster, T. (2009). Dogs in society can prevent society going to the dogs. *The Veterinary Journal*, 179(3), 322–323.

Mills, D. & Hall, S. (2014). Animal-assisted interventions: making better use of the human–animal bond. *Veterinary Record*, 174(11), 269–273.

Mintel (2011). *Pet Food and Supplies – UK: Mintel Marketing Report*. Mintel International, London.

Moody, W.J., King, R. & O'Rourke, S.O. (2002). Attitudes of paediatric medical ward staff to a dog visitation programme. *Journal of Clinical Nursing*, 11(4), 537–544.

Mugford, R.A. & M'Comisky, J.G. (1975). Some recent work on the psychotherapeutic value of cage birds with elderly people. In R.S. Anderson (Ed.), *Pet Animals and Society*. Baillere Tindal, London, pp. 54–65.

Murray, J.K., Browne, J.W., Roberts, A.M., Whitmarsh, A. & Gruffydd-Jones, J.T. (2010). Number and ownership profiles of cats and dogs in the UK. *Veterinary Record*, 166, 163–168.

Murray, J.K., Gruffydd-Jones, T.J., Roberts, M.A. & Browne, W.J. (2015). Assessing changes in the UK pet cat and dog populations: numbers and household ownership. *Veterinary Record*, 177(10), 259.

National Literacy Trust (2009). Manifesto for literacy. Available at: http://www.literacytrust.org.uk/assets/0000/2584/manifestoforliteracyfullversion.pdf (accessed 31 May 2016).

Oberle, D., Mutius, E.V. & Kries, R.V. (2003). Childhood asthma and continuous exposure to cats since the first year of life with cats allowed in the child's bedroom. *Allergy*, 58(10), 1033–1036.

Odendaal, J.S.J. (2000). Animal-assisted therapy – magic or medicine? *Journal of Psychosomatic Research*, 49(4), 275–280.

Office for National Statistics (ONS) (2013). Statistical bulletin: Families and households 2013. Available at: http://www.ons.gov.uk/peoplepopulationandcommunity/birthsdeathsandmarriages/families/bulletins/familiesandhouseholds/2013-10-31 (accessed 31 May 2016).

O'Haire, M. (2010). Companion animals and human health: benefits, challenges, and the road ahead. *Journal of Veterinary Behavior: Clinical Applications and Research*, 5(5), 226–234.

Oka, K. & Shibata, A. (2009). Dog ownership and health-related physical activity among Japanese adults. *Journal of Physical Activity and Health*, 6(4), 412–418.

Orritt, R. (2014). Dog ownership has unknown risks but known health benefits: we need evidence based policy. *BMJ*, 349, 4081.

Owen, C.G., Nightingale, C.M., Rudnicka, A.R., Ekelund, U., McMinn, A.M., van Sluijis, E.M., Cook, D.G. & Whincup, P.H. (2010). Family dog ownership and levels of physical activity in childhood: findings from the Child Heart and Health Study in England. *American Journal of Public Health*, 100(9), 1669–1671.

Ownby, D., Johnson, C. & Peterson, E. (2002). Exposure to dogs and cats in the first year of life and risk of allergic sensitization at 6 to 7 years of age. *Journal of the American Medical Association*, 288, 963–972.

Pederson, I., Martinsen, E.W., Berget, B. & Braastad, B.O. (2012). Farm animal-assisted intervention for people with clinical depression: a randomised controlled task. *Anthrozoös*, 25, 149–160.

Peretti, P.O. (1990). Elderly–animal friendship bonds. *Social Behavior and Personality: An International Journal*, 18(1), 151–156.

Perzanowski, M.S., Rönmark, E., Platts-Mills, T.A. & Lundbäck, B. (2002). Effect of cat and dog ownership on sensitization and development of asthma among pre-teenage children. *American Journal of Respiratory and Critical Care Medicine*, 166(5), 696–702.

Pet Business World (2016). UK pet food market reaches £2.8 billion. Available at: http://www.petbusinessworld.co.uk/news/feed/uk-pet-food-market-reaches--2-8-billion (accessed 31 May 2016).

Pet Food Manufacturers Association (PFMA) (2014). Pet obesity: Five years on. Available at: http://www.pfma.org.uk/_assets/docs/PFMA_WhitePaper_2014.pdf (accessed 31 May 2016).

Pet Food Manufacturers Association (PFMA) (2015). Pet Population 2015. Available at: http://www.pfma.org.uk/pet-population-2015 (accessed 7 February 2016).

Pets in the Classroom (2015). Benefits of classroom animals. Available at: http://www.petsintheclassroom.org/teachers/benefits-of-classroom-animals/ (accessed 31 May 2016).

Philips, C. (2002). Does pet ownership reduce the number of GP consultations? What pets can do for patients. Presented at 'Pets are Good for People', a meeting of the Comparative Medicine Section, Royal Society of Medicine, London.

Platts-Mills T., Vaughan, J., Squillace, S., Woodfolk, J. & Sporik, R. (2001). Sensitisation, asthma, and a modified Th2 response in children exposed to cat allergen: a population-based cross-sectional study. *The Lancet*, 357(9258), 752–756.

Prince's Trust (2007). The Cost of Exclusion: Counting the cost of youth disadvantage in the UK. Available at: http://intouniversity.org/sites/all/files/userfiles/files/Prince's%20Trust%20Cost%20of%20youth%20exclusion.pdf (accessed 15 September 2016).

Qureshi, A.I., Memon, M.Z., Vazquez, G. & Suri, M.F.K. (2009). Cat ownership and the risk of fatal cardiovascular diseases. Results from the Second National Health and Nutrition Examination Study Mortality Follow-up Study. *Journal of Vascular and Interventional Neurology*, 2(1), 132.

Raina, P., Bonnett, B. & Waltner-Toews, D. (1998). Relationship between pet ownership and healthcare among seniors. Presented at the 8th International Conference on Human–Animal Interactions, 'The Changing Roles of Animals in Society', Prague, Czech Republic, September 1998.

Ramos, D. & Mills, D.S. (2009). Human directed aggression in Brazilian domestic cats: owner reported prevalence, contexts and risk factors. *Journal of Feline Medicine and Surgery*, 11(10), 835–841.

Rieger, G. & Turner, D.C. (1999). How depressive moods affect the behavior of singly living persons toward their cats. *Anthrozoös*, 12(4), 224–233.

Royal Mail Group (2012). Inquiry into dog attacks on postal workers. Available at: http://www.royalmailgroup.com/sites/default/files/Langley_Report.pdf (accessed 31 May 2016).

Royal National Institute for the Blind (RNIB) (2013). Sight loss UK 2013. Available at: http://www.rnib.org.uk/sites/default/files/Sight_loss_UK_2013.pdf (accessed 31 May 2016).

Sainsbury, M. & Schagen, I. (2004). Attitudes to reading at ages nine and eleven. *Journal of Research in Reading*, 27(4), 373–386.

Salmon, I.M., Hogarth-Scott, R.S. & Lavelle, R.B. (1982). A dog in residence: the JACOPIS study. *The Latham Letter*. The Latham Foundation, Alaceda, California.

Salmon, J. (2007). Do families with pets have more active children? In *Proceedings of People, Pets and Planning Symposium: Living in a Healthy Community*. Deakin University, Melbourne, Australia, November 2007, pp. 23–25.

Salmon, J., Timperio, A., Chu, B. & Veitch, J. (2010). Dog ownership, dog walking, and children's and parents' physical activity. *Research Quarterly for Exercise and Sport*, 81(3), 264–271.

Salmon, P.W. & Salmon, I.M. (1983). Who owns you? Psychological research into the human–pet bond in Australia. In A.H. Katcher & A.M. Beck (Eds), *New Perspectives on our Lives with Companion Animals*. University of Pennsylvania Press, Philadelphia, Pennsylvania, pp. 244–265.

Sellers, D.M. (2006). The evaluation of an animal assisted therapy intervention for elders with dementia in long-term care. *Activities, Adaptation and Aging*, 30(1), 61–77.

Serpell, J.A. (1983). The personality of the dog and its influence on the pet–owner bond. In A.H. Katcher & A.M. Beck (Eds), *New Perspectives on our Lives with Companion Animals*. University of Pennsylvania Press, Philadelphia, Pennsylvania, pp. 57–63.

Serpell, J.A. (1990). Evidence for long term effects of pet ownership on human health. *Pets, Benefits and Practice*, 20, 1–7.

Serpell, J.A. (1991). Beneficial effects of pet ownership on some aspects of human health and behaviour. *Journal of the Royal Society of Medicine*, 84(12), 717–720.

Shaw, D.M. (2013). Man's best friend as a reading facilitator? *The Reading Teacher*, 66, 365–371.

Siegel, J.M. (1990). Stressful life events and use of physician services among the elderly: the moderating role of pet ownership. *Journal of Personality and Social Psychology*, 58, 1081–1086.

Siegel, J.M. (1995). Pet ownership and the importance of pets among adolescents. *Anthrozoös*, 8(4), 217–223.

Siegel, K., Karus, D. & Raveis, V.H. (1996). Adjustment of children facing the death of a parent due to cancer. *Journal of the American Academy of Child & Adolescent Psychiatry*, 35(4), 442–450.

Siegel, J.M., Angulo, F.J., Detels, R., Wesch, J. & Mullen, A. (1999). AIDS diagnosis and depression in the Multi-center AIDS Cohort Study: the ameliorating impact of pet ownership. *AIDS Care*, 11(2), 157–170.

Statista (2015). Estimated lifetime cost of keeping pet dogs, cats and rabbits in the United Kingdom (UK) as of 2015 (in 1,000 GBP). Available at: http://www.statista.com/statistics/299910/lifetime-cost-of-dogs-cats-and-rabbit-pets-in-the-united-kingdom-uk/ (accessed 20 June 2016).

Straede, C.M. & Gates, R.G. (1993). Psychological health in a population of Australian cat owners. *Anthrozoös*, 6(1), 30–42.

Support Dogs (n.d.). About us. Available at: http://www.support-dogs.org.uk/about-us/our-dogs (accessed 3 September 2016).

Taking Part Survey (2009/10). Taking part – statistical release. Available at: https://www.gov.uk/government/uploads/system/uploads/attachment_data/file/77322/TakingPart_AdultChild2009-10_StatisticalRelease.pdf (accessed 31 May 2016).

The Kennel Club (2016). Case studies: Abbie and Spike. Available at: http://www.thekennelclub.org.uk/our-resources/kennel-club-campaigns/bark-and-read/case-studies-abbie-and-spike (accessed 31 May 2016).

The Pet Site (2014). More cats being abandoned than ever before. Available at: http://www.thepetsite.co.uk/news/13836/more-cats-being-abandoned-than-ever-before/ (accessed 31 May 2016).

The Telegraph (2014). Dog attack laws and statistics. Available at: http://www.telegraph.co.uk/news/uknews/law-and-order/10429862/Dog-attack-laws-and-statistics.html (accessed 31 May 2016).

Thorpe, R.J., Simonsick, E.M., Brach, J.S., Ayonayou, H., Satterfield, S., Harris, T.B., Garcia, M. & Kritchevsky, S.B. (2006). Dog ownership, walking behavior, and maintained mobility in late life. *Journal of the American Geriatrics Society*, 54(9), 1419–1424.

Timperio, A., Salmon, J., Chu, B. & Andrianopoulos, N. (2008). Is dog ownership or dog walking associated with weight status in children and their parents? *Health Promotion Journal of Australia*, 19(1), 60–63.

Turner, D.C., Rieger, G. & Gygax, L. (2003). Spouses and cats and their effects on human mood. *Anthrozoös*, 16(3), 213–228.

UK Public Spending (2013). Public spending details for 2013. Available at: http://www.ukpublicspending.co.uk/year_spending_2013UKbn_13bc1n_10#ukgs302 (accessed 31 May 2016).

Upton, V. (2005). Dogs: a potential public health role to improve health and well-being. *The SCAS Journal*, 17(3), 2–5.

US Department of Health and Human Services (1996). *Physical Activity and Health: a Report of the Surgeon General*. US Department of Health and Human Services, Centers for Disease Control and Prevention, National Center for Chronic Disease Prevention and Health Promotion. Available at: https://www.cdc.gov/nccdphp/sgr/pdf/sgrfull.pdf (accessed 2 September 2016).

Vet Times (2015). 47,000 dogs abandoned in past year, Dogs Trust survey reveals. Available at: http://www.vettimes.co.uk/news/47000-dogs-abandoned-in-past-year-dogs-trust-survey-reveals/ (accessed 31 May 2016).

Vormbrock, J.K. & Grossberg, J.M. (1988). Cardiovascular effects of human–pet dog interactions. *Journal of Behaviour Medicine*, 11(5), 509–517.

Wells, D.L. (2009). The effects of animals on human health and well-being. *Journal of Social Issues*, 65(3), 523–543.

Westgarth, C., Liu, J., Heron, J., Ness, A.R., Bundred, P., Gaskell, R.M., German, A.J., McCune, S. & Dawson, S. (2012). Dog ownership during pregnancy, maternal activity, and obesity: a cross-sectional study. *PLoS ONE*, 7(2), e31315.

Westgarth, C., Boddy, L.M., Stratton, G., German, A.J., Gaskell, R.M., Coyne, K.P., Bundred, P., McCune, S. & Dawson, S. (2013). Pet ownership, dog types and attachment to pets in 9–10 year old children in Liverpool, UK. *BMC Veterinary Research*, 9, 102.

Wilson, C.C. (1991). The pet as an anxiolytic intervention. *Journal of Nervous Mental Disorders*, 179, 482–489.

Wood, L., Martin, K., Christian, H., Nathan, A., Lauritsen, C., Houghton, S., Kawachi, I. & McCune, S. (2015). The pet factor – companion animals as a conduit for getting to know people, friendship formation and social support. *PLoS ONE* 10(4): e0122085.

World Health Organization (1946). WHO definition of Health. Available at: http://www.who.int/about/definition/en/print.html (accessed 31 May 2016).

Wright, J.C. & Moore, D. (1982). Comments on animal companions and one-year survival of patients after discharge from a coronary care unit. *Public Health Reports*, 97(4), 380–381.

Wright, H., Hall, S., Hames, A., Hardiman, J., Mills, R., PAWS Team & Mills, D. (2015a). Pet dogs improve family functioning and reduce anxiety in children with autism spectrum disorder. *Anthrozoös*, 28(4), 611–624.

Wright, H.F., Hall, S., Hames, A., Hardiman, J., Mills, R., PAWS Team & Mills, D.S. (2015b). Acquiring a pet dog significantly reduces stress of primary carers for children with autism spectrum disorder: a prospective case control study. *Journal of Autism and Developmental Disorders*, 45(8), 2531–2540.

Wright, H.F., Hall, S. & Mills, D.S. (2016). Additional evidence is needed to recommend acquiring a dog to families of children with autism spectrum disorder: a response to Crossman and Kazdin. *Journal of Autism and Developmental Disorders*, 46, 336–339.

Zasloff, R.L. & Kidd, A.H. (1994). Loneliness and pet ownership among single women. *Psychological Reports*, 75, 747–752.

Zimolag, U.U. & Krupa, T. (2009). Pet ownership as a meaningful community occupation for people with serious mental illness. *American Journal of Occupational Therapy*, 63(2), 126–137.

Index

Page numbers in **bold** refer to figures and tables.

welfare, animal 15, 17
wheelchair users, assistance
            dogs 50–51
Wood Green Animal Shelter 6, 21
working animals 1, 2
    see also assistance dogs
World Health Organization,
            'health' definition 34

Yellow Pages™ 4, 11
You and Yours (Radio 4
            documentaries) 7
youth unemployment 53–54

zoonotic diseases 15, 22